Contemporary Diagnosis
and Management of

Allergic
Diseases
and Asthma®

James E. Gern, MD
Professor of Pediatrics

University of Wisconsin-Madison
Medical School

William W. Busse, MD
Professor of Medicine

University of Wisconsin-Madison
Medical School

Fourth Edition

D0862604

Published by
Handbooks in Health Care Co.,
a division of Associates in Medical Marketing Co., Inc.
Newtown, Pennsylvania, USA

Acknowledgements

The authors thank Yvonne Gern for word processing and preparation of tables and figures.

International Standard Book Number: 1-884065-83-X

Library of Congress Catalog Card Number: 2002116832

Contents

This book has been prepared and is presented as a service to the medical community. The information provided reflects the knowledge, experience, and personal opinions of William W. Busse, MD, Professor of Medicine, and James E. Gern, MD, Professor of Pediatrics, University of Wisconsin-Madison Medical School, Madison, Wisconsin.

This book is not intended to replace or to be used as a substitute for the complete prescribing information prepared by each manufacturer for each drug. Because of possible variations in drug indications, in dosage information, in newly described toxicities, in drug interactions, and in other items of importance, reference to such complete prescribing information is definitely recommended before any of the drugs discussed are used or prescribed.

1

The Epidemiology
of Allergic Diseases

Asthma, allergic rhinitis, food allergy, and atopic dermatitis tend to occur in the same families and even in the same individuals. These clinical observations have prompted detailed analysis of the epidemiology of these related disorders and have led to new insights into common and unique pathologic mechanisms, the natural history of these disorders, and the development of new preventive and therapeutic strategies. This chapter reviews the epidemiology of common allergic disorders, including prevalence, risk factors, and natural history, and examines possible causes for recent increases in allergy-related morbidity and mortality.

Role of Genetics and the Environment in the Pathogenesis of Allergy

Atopy, or the propensity to produce allergen-specific or increased total immunoglobulin E (IgE), is a common component of atopic diseases such as asthma, allergic rhinitis, food allergy, and atopic dermatitis (Figure 1). Although most patients with asthma or allergic rhinitis produce allergen-specific IgE, some patients have similar clinical manifestations despite having negative skin tests or radioallergosorbent tests. The mechanism for chronic

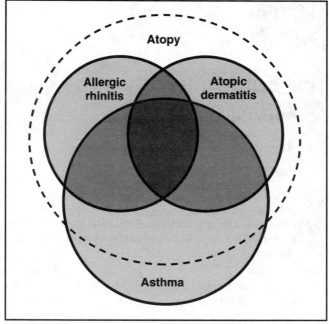

Figure 1: Relationship of atopy and allergic diseases.

skin or airway inflammation without demonstrable allergy is unknown.

Another pathogenic factor common to allergic disorders is chronic inflammation involving mast cells, basophils, T cells, and eosinophils. Many of the genes for the cytokines and receptors that regulate allergic inflammation are clustered on a short segment of chromosome 5q, and linkage of total serum IgE levels to these genes has been demonstrated in some families.[1] In contrast, production of IgE specific for many of the common pollen and pet allergens has been linked to certain class II HLA molecules.[2] These data indicate that the inheritance of allergic disorders is multifactorial. Furthermore, additional factors apparently influence whether a person born into an atopic family will develop allergic rhinitis, asthma, atopic dermatitis, or some combination of these disorders. For example, Dold and colleagues[3] found that families with one parent who had atopic dermatitis were more likely to have a child with atopic dermatitis (odds ratio [OR] 3.4) than were families with one parent with either asthma (OR 1.5) or allergic rhinitis (OR 1.4). Similar trends were observed when inherited asthma or atopic dermatitis was examined, suggesting that additional genetic and environmental factors influence which organ system(s) is affected by allergy. In support of this concept, genes within chromosome 5q and elsewhere have been linked to the development of bronchial hyperresponsiveness, a key feature of asthma.[4,5]

Although genetics is an important determinant of allergy, environmental exposures undoubtedly contribute to the variability in the expression of allergic diseases in atopic individuals. Environmental factors that may influence the development of allergy include allergen exposure, indoor and/or outdoor air pollution, childhood infections, family size, and rural vs urban lifestyle. The effects of allergen exposure on the development of allergy have been measured prospectively. Infants who are either breast-fed by mothers who restrict their intake of allergenic foods or fed hypoallergenic protein hydrolysate formulas for the first few months of life have a decreased incidence of food allergy and atopic dermatitis, although the incidence of respiratory allergy is unchanged.[6-8] Furthermore, respiratory allergy is more likely to develop in children who are exposed early in life to high levels of indoor allergens such as house dust mites.[9] Adults may also develop respiratory allergy when exposed to a new allergen, and this has been demonstrated in an epidemiologic study of an asthma outbreak in New Guinea.[10] In this case, bringing blankets into the homes led to a sharp increase in exposure to house dust mite proteins, and the development of mite-specific IgE was strongly associated with the onset of asthma. Exposure to new allergens in the workplace can also lead to the development of new-onset allergic rhinitis, dermatitis, or asthma in previously healthy adults.[11]

The relationship between animal exposure and allergy has recently been reevaluated. It is clear that pet ownership increases symptoms of respiratory allergy and asthma in people who are allergic to their pets. Recently, however, several studies have demonstrated that having a pet in the home during infancy actually reduces the risk of developing allergy. These results imply that there may be unique mechanisms for developing immune tolerance to allergens in infancy, although these mechanisms have yet to be clearly defined.

The recognition of the high prevalence of respiratory allergy in inner-city neighborhoods such as those in Chicago and New York City has refocused attention on the potential role of air pollution in allergy pathogenesis. Most of the data, however, indicate that while outdoor pollutants such as ozone, NO_2, and diesel particles are important triggers of acute respiratory symptoms,[12] exposure to them is unlikely to cause asthma.[13] More convincing data link the development of asthma to indoor air pollutants such as tobacco smoke. Active or passive exposure to smoke is associated with an increased incidence of many respiratory disorders, including asthma and allergic rhinitis.[6,14] Exposure to irritants generated by gas stoves or other indoor sources of combustion has also been associated with increased respiratory symptoms and asthma.[15]

The effects of lower respiratory infections in infancy on the subsequent risk for asthma and allergen sensitization have also been prospectively examined. Contracting a wheezy lower respiratory infection (bronchiolitis) at an early age increases the risk of developing additional wheezing illnesses in infancy.[16] In addition, infants with recurrent bronchiolitis who go on to develop allergen-specific IgE are at increased risk for developing typical allergic asthma in childhood.[17] Whether bronchiolitis itself increases the risk of developing asthma is controversial, although long-term, prospective studies suggest that both pneumonia and respiratory syncytial virus bronchiolitis in infancy are associated with increased risk of asthma in childhood.[18,19]

In summary, these epidemiologic studies indicate that allergic disorders overlap in clinical expression, genetic linkage, and pathogenic mechanisms. Despite these similarities, genetic and environmental factors likely influence the severity and target organ specificity of allergic disorders.

Incidence, Prevalence, and Natural History of Allergic Disorders
Asthma

According to the United States National Health Interview Study (NHIS), the prevalence of asthma rose from 31 per 1,000 population in 1980 to 54 per 1,000 during 1993-1994.[20] This 74% increase in asthma prevalence is representative of trends in other developed countries. Asthma is one of the leading causes for outpatient health-care visits and hospitalizations,[21] accounting for a financial burden estimated to exceed $4 billion per year in the United States alone. Other costs attributable to asthma include huge losses from lost workdays, limitations in activity, and psychological stress. Finally, after decades of declining death rates from asthma, mortality increased an average of 6.2% a year during the 1980s.[22]

Asthma prevalence and morbidity are not evenly distributed. Worldwide, developed countries have much higher levels of asthma than do Third World countries.[23] In the United States, children, minorities, and inner-city residents are disproportionately affected and have experienced the greatest increase in prevalence and death rates in recent years.[13,20,22,24]

Asthma usually begins during early childhood, and most children have their first episode of asthma before their third birthday.[25] Atopic dermatitis and the development of elevated total or allergen-specific IgE during infancy indicate increased risk for subsequent asthma.[26] Asthma prevalence is strongly related to atopy and especially to positive skin tests

9

for house dust mite, *Alternaria,* cockroach, or cat.[27,28] Seventy-five percent to 85% of asthma patients have positive skin reactions to allergies, and there is a strong correlation between the number of positive skin tests in children and the severity of asthma.[29,30] Up to half of asthmatic children will no longer be symptomatic as adults, and the absence of eczema or allergic rhinitis is a good prognostic indicator.[21,31] Children with severe asthma, however, are likely to continue to have problems as adults.

Allergy is also a contributing factor in most adults with asthma and can involve the same spectrum of allergens associated with asthma in children. Exposure to airborne allergens or chemicals in the working environment should also be considered in evaluating an adult with asthma.[11] Despite the difference in triggers for allergic and nonallergic asthma, the character of the airway inflammation and clinical manifestations are similar. Most adults with asthma had the onset of their respiratory complaints in childhood, or, less often, in the 2nd through the 4th decades. Middle-aged or elderly patients with a new onset of symptoms that suggest asthma should be carefully evaluated for other disorders in the differential diagnosis, such as chronic obstructive pulmonary disease, mechanical obstruction of the airway, gastroesophageal reflux, chronic infections with mycoplasma or chlamydia, or respiratory complaints of cardiac origin. In general, adult-onset asthma is less likely to resolve spontaneously than asthma that begins in childhood.

Allergic rhinitis

Allergic rhinitis is the most common manifestation of atopy, affecting up to 20% of the population, and is the sixth most prevalent health problem in the United States.[32] Allergic rhinitis thus has a significant impact on public health and accounts for huge expenditures for prescription and over-the-counter medications. Complications associated with allergic rhinitis include loss of taste and smell, sleep disorders, sinusitis, eustachian tube dysfunction, otitis media,[33] and facial growth abnormalities such as overbite.

Risk factors for the development of allergic rhinitis include asthma, family history of allergy, persistent sensitization to foods in infancy, elevated serum IgE, and exposure to cigarette smoke and environmental allergens.[15,20,34] Chronic rhinitis from sensitization to perennial allergens such as house dust mite and pet danders can develop in infancy, while rhinitis triggered by seasonal pollen allergens begins to appear in school-age children. The peak prevalence of allergic rhinitis occurs in the teen years or early 20s, and symptoms typically become milder in middle age. Approximately 20% of children with allergic rhinitis eventually become asymptomatic, although other manifestations of atopy, such as asthma, may persist.

Atopic dermatitis

Atopic dermatitis is often the first manifestation of allergy in an atopic child, and approximately 80% of cases begin before the age of 3 years.[35] It is especially common in children and adolescents. Estimates of cumulative prevalence range from 9% to 21% in childhood, while prevalence in adults is estimated to be 2% to 10%.[36,37] As is the case with other common allergic disorders, the prevalence of atopic dermatitis has increased in the past 30 years.[38] The prevalence of atopic dermatitis can be markedly different in similar ethnic populations living in different geographic regions, indicating that environmental factors are important in determining disease expression.[39] The prognosis for atopic dermatitis is generally favorable, and symptoms abate completely in about one third of cases that begin during childhood.

Atopic dermatitis is often associated with other allergic disorders and with overproduction of IgE. In a prospective study of newborns in Tucson, cord blood IgE levels were related to the subsequent incidence of atopic dermatitis.[40] The development of food allergy can also significantly affect the severity of atopic dermatitis. One third to one half of children referred to tertiary-care allergy clinics for severe atopic dermatitis have underlying food allergy.[41,42] Eliminating the of-

11

fending food from the diet can significantly improve the skin condition, as well as coexistent rhinitis and asthma.[41,43]

Atopic dermatitis in adults is rarely aggravated by food allergy, but occupational exposures frequently contribute to disease severity.[44] Atopic individuals have a much greater incidence of occupational dermatitis, which most commonly affects the hands. Precipitants of occupational dermatitis include irritants and allergens. Careful review of working conditions, household chores, and hobbies often identifies likely antagonists and suggests effective avoidance measures. Nonetheless, occupational dermatitis remains a major cause of work-related disability.

Why Are Atopic Diseases Increasing in Prevalence and Severity?

Asthma, atopic dermatitis, and allergic rhinitis are all increasing in prevalence, even after accounting for time-related differences in diagnostic criteria. These trends, plus the much greater prevalence of allergy in developed vs Third World countries,[39] raise the possibility that the causative factors are linked to changes in lifestyles associated with modern industrial society. The underlying reasons to explain the increase in atopic diseases are the subject of intense research, and a number of theories have been proposed.

In the United States, the inner-city environment is associated with particularly high rates of asthma, surpassing 50% in some neighborhoods, and this has prompted a large, multicenter study to identify the causative factors.[45] Allergen exposure can be very high, and the allergy most closely associated with asthma in the inner city is the cockroach. The effect of outdoor air pollution on asthma has also been extensively evaluated. Clearly, polluted air can trigger symptoms in people who already have asthma, but so far there is no clear link between air pollution and increased asthma prevalence.[13]

One of the changes associated with modern lifestyles in Western countries is reduced exposure to infectious disease and, probably, reduced exposure to microorganisms in general. One theory, dubbed 'the hygiene hypothesis,' states that routine exposure to microorganisms helps the immune system to develop normally; if this exposure does not occur, the risk for allergic diseases is increased. In support of this hypothesis, the number of older siblings in the family, which presumably determines the exposures to infectious diseases in early childhood, is inversely related to the odds of allergen sensitization.[46] Although the mechanisms for these effects are unknown, some researchers speculate that frequent respiratory infections during childhood stimulate interferon-γ production and that increased amounts of this cytokine during a critical stage of immune system development might reduce the risk of developing allergic diseases.[47] Using a similar line of reasoning, it has also been postulated that increased exposure to bacteria in an agrarian environment might protect against allergy. Finally, some data suggest that antibiotic use and lack of breast-feeding change the intestinal microflora in such a way to increase the risk of allergy.[48] Each of these hypotheses is thought-provoking, but additional studies are needed to determine which have clinical merit.

Asthma is increasing not only in frequency, but also in severity, especially in children, minorities, and patients from urban centers.[20] Reasons for these trends appear to be multifactorial and include environmental factors (see above), socioeconomic factors such as access to health care and the ability to purchase asthma medications, underuse of anti-inflammatory medications, and attitudes related to health issues in general. The challenge is to determine which of these factors are important in asthma pathogenesis in individual patient populations so that remedial resources can be mobilized and targeted appropriately.

Summary

Epidemiologic studies have provided important insight into the fundamental issues related to allergic diseases, including determining the contributions of genetics and the environment to pathogenesis and defining the recent trends toward increasing prevalence and severity. Future studies involving high-risk populations will likely identify the principal factors driving these trends and thus enable the creation of better strategies for the prevention and treatment of allergic disorders.

References

1. Barnes KC: Evidence for common genetic elements in allergic disease. *J Allergy Clin Immunol* 2000;106:S192-S200.

2. Howell WM, Holgate ST: HLA genetics and allergic disease. *Thorax* 1995;50:815-818.

3. Dold S, Wjst M, von Mutius E, et al: Genetic risk for asthma, allergic rhinitis, and atopic dermatitis. *Arch Dis Child* 1992; 67:1018-1022.

4. Postma DS, Bleecker ER, Amelung PJ, et al: Genetic susceptibility to asthma—bronchial hyperresponsiveness coinherited with a major gene for atopy. *N Engl J Med* 1995;333:894-900.

5. De Sanctis GT, Merchant M, Beier DR, et al: Quantitative locus analysis of airway hyperresponsiveness in A/J and C57BL/6J mice. *Nat Genet* 1995;11:150-154.

6. Zeiger RS, Heller S: The development and prediction of atopy in high-risk children: follow-up at age seven years in a prospective randomized study of combined maternal and infant food allergen avoidance. *J Allergy Clin Immunol* 1995;95:1179-1190.

7. Sigurs N, Hattevig G, Kjellman B: Maternal avoidance of eggs, cow's milk, and fish during lactation: effect on allergic manifestations, skin-prick tests, and specific IgE antibodies in children at age 4 years. *Pediatrics* 1992;89:735-739.

8. Mallet E, Henocq A: Long-term prevention of allergic diseases by using protein hydrolysate formula in at-risk infants. *J Pediatr* 1992;121:S95-S100.

9. Platts-Mills TA, Vaughan JW, Carter MC, et al: The risk of intervention in established allergy: avoidance of indoor allergens in the treatment of chronic allergic disease. *J Allergy Clin Immunol* 2000;106:787-804.

10. Dowse GK, Turner KJ, Stewart GA, et al: The association between *Dermatophagoides* mites and the increasing prevalence

of asthma in village communities within the Papua New Guinea Highlands. *J Allergy Clin Immunol* 1985;75:75-83.

11. Chan-Yeung M, Malo JL: Occupational asthma. *N Engl J Med* 1995;333:107-112.

12. Committee of the Environmental and Occupational Health Assembly of the American Thoracic Society: Health effects of outdoor air pollution. *Am J Respir Crit Care Med* 1996;153:3-50.

13. Koren HS, Utell MJ: Asthma and the environment. *Eur Health Perspectives* 1997;105:534-537.

14. Martinez FD, Cline M, Burrows B: Increased incidence of asthma in children of smoking mothers. *Pediatrics* 1992;89:21-26.

15. Ostro BD, Lipsett MJ, Mann JK, et al: Indoor air pollution and asthma. Results from a panel study. *Am J Respir Crit Care Med* 1994;149:1400-1406.

16. Morgan WJ, Martinez FD: Risk factors for developing wheezing and asthma in childhood. *Pediatr Clin North Am* 1992;39:1185-1203.

17. Martinez FD, Wright AL, Taussig LM, et al: Asthma and wheezing in the first six years of life. The Group Health Medical Associates. *N Engl J Med* 1995; 332:133-138.

18. Castro-Rodríguez JA, et al: Association of radiologically ascertained pneumonia before age 3 yr with asthmalike symptoms and pulmonary function during childhood. *Crit Care Med* 1999;159:1891-1897.

19. Stein RT, et al: Respiratory syncytial virus in early life and risk of wheeze and allergy by age 13 years. *Lancet* 1999; 354:541-545.

20. Centers for Disease Control and Prevention: Surveillance for asthma—United States, 1960-1995. *MMWR* 1998;47:1-26.

21. Taylor WR, Newacheck PW: Impact of childhood asthma on health. *Pediatrics* 1992;90:657-662.

22. Weiss KB, Wagener DK: Changing patterns of asthma mortality. Identifying target populations at high risk. *JAMA* 1990; 264:1683-1687.

23. Evans R 3rd: Asthma among minority children. A growing problem. *Chest* 1992;101:368S-371S.

24. Lang DM, Polansky M: Patterns of asthma mortality in Philadelphia from 1969 to 1991. *N Engl J Med* 1994;331: 1542-1546.

25. Gergen PJ, Mullally DI, Evans R 3rd: National survey of prevalence of asthma among children in the United States, 1976 to 1980. *Pediatrics* 1988;81:1-7.

26. ETAC Study Group: Allergic factors associated with the development of asthma and the influence of cetirizine in a double-blind, randomized, placebo-controlled trial: first results of ETAC. *Pediatr Allergy Immunol* 1998;9:116-124.

27. Rosenstreich DL, Eggleston PA, Kattan M, et al: The role of cockroach allergy and exposure to cockroach allergen in causing morbidity among inner-city children with asthma. *N Engl J Med* 1997;336:1356-1363.

28. Gergen PJ, Turkeltaub PC: The association of individual allergen reactivity with respiratory disease in a national sample: data from the second National Health and Nutrition Examination Survey, 1976-80 (NHANES II). *J Allergy Clin Immunol* 1992;90: 579-588.

29. Martin AJ, Landau LI, Phelan PD: Natural history of allergy in asthmatic children followed to adult life. *Med J Aust* 1981;2: 470-474.

30. Zimmerman B, Chambers C, Forsyth S: Allergy in asthma. II. The highly atopic infant and chronic asthma. *J Allergy Clin Immunol* 1988;81:71-77.

31. Aberg N: Asthma and allergic rhinitis in Swedish conscripts. *Clin Exp Allergy* 1989;19:59-63.

32. Collins JG: *Prevalence of Selected Chronic Conditions, United States, 1983-85.* National Center for Health Statistics; DHHS publication No. (PHS) 88-1250,1988.

33. Naclerio RM: Allergic rhinitis. *N Engl J Med* 1991;325: 860-869.

34. Kulig M, et al: Long-lasting sensitization to food during the first two years precedes allergic airway disease. *Pediatr Allergy Immunol* 1998;9:61-67.

35. Leung DY: Atopic dermatitis: the skin as a window into the pathogenesis of chronic allergic diseases. *J Allergy Clin Immunol* 1995;96:302-318.

36. Croner S: Atopic dermatitis—epidemiology. *Pediatr Allergy Immunol* 1991;2:6-7.

37. Johnson ML, Johnson KG, Engel A: Prevalence, morbidity, and cost of dermatologic diseases. *J Am Acad Dermatol* 1984; 11:930-936.

38. Williams HC: Is the prevalence of atopic eczema rising? *Clin Exp Dermatol* 1992;17:385-391.

39. Williams H, et al: Worldwide variations in the prevalence of symptoms of atopic eczema in the international study of asthma and allergies in childhood. *J Allergy Clin Immunol* 1999;103:125-138.

40. Halonen M, Stern D, Taussig LM, et al: The predictive relationship between serum IgE levels at birth and subsequent incidences of lower respiratory illnesses and eczema in infants. *Am Rev Respir Dis* 1992;146:866-870.

41. Sampson HA, McCaskill CC: Food hypersensitivity and atopic dermatitis: evaluation of 113 patients. *J Pediatr* 1985; 107:669-675.

42. Jones SM, Sampson HA: The role of allergens in atopic dermatitis. *Clin Rev Allergy* 1993;11:471-490.

43. James JM, Bernhisel-Broadbent J, Sampson HA: Respiratory reactions provoked by double-blind food challenges in children. *Am J Respir Crit Care Med* 1994;149:59-64.

44. Rystedt I: Work-related hand eczema in atopics. *Contact Dermatitis* 1985;12:164-171.

45. Eggleston PA, et al: Relationship of indoor allergic exposure to skin test sensitivity in inner-city children with asthma. *J Allergy Clin Immunol* 1998;102:563-570.

46. Strachan DP, Harkins LS, Johnston ID, et al: Childhood antecedents of allergic sensitization in young British adults. *J Allergy Clin Immunol* 1997;99:6-12.

47. Shaheen SO: Changing patterns of childhood infection and the rise in allergic disease. *Clin Exp Allergy* 1995;25:1034-1037.

48. Bjorksten B, et al: The intestinal microflora in allergic Estonian and Swedish 2-year-old children. *Clin Exp Allergy* 1999;29:342-346.

2

Differential Diagnosis of Allergic Diseases and Asthma

Allergic disorders can involve the skin, respiratory tract, gastrointestinal tract, cardiovascular system, and even the central nervous system and can thereby cause a wide variety of signs and symptoms. Because allergic diseases are common and varied in their presentation, clinicians need to have a clear understanding of the diagnostic features of allergic disorders and to be able to differentiate allergy from other diseases that present in a similar fashion. For example, although the onset of chronic nasal congestion during the pollen season usually indicates allergic rhinitis, it is important to recognize the patient whose congested nose is an indication of a less common problem, such as a systemic illness (eg, hypothyroidism), a nasal polyp, or cocaine abuse. Not considering the differential diagnosis can lead to delays in appropriate therapy. Conversely, overdiagnosis of allergic disorders can lead to inappropriate or unnecessary prescribed therapy. For example, prescribing an overly restrictive diet for a child who has been mistakenly diagnosed as having food allergy may lead to nutritional deficiencies.

This chapter provides a quick reference to the diagnostic criteria and differential diagnosis for asthma and the most common allergic disorders. Subsequent chapters examine additional information about the diagnostic and therapeutic approaches to allergic disorders.

Allergic Conjunctivitis
Diagnostic features
Allergic conjunctivitis, also known as hay fever conjunctivitis, is immunoglobulin E (IgE)-mediated inflammation of the conjunctiva triggered by outdoor allergens, such as pollen or mold, or indoor allergens, such as pet dander or house dust mite. Symptoms include itching, redness, and tearing of the eyes, often accompanied by swelling of the periocular tissues. One of the cardinal features of allergic rhinoconjunctivitis is the coexistence of allergic rhinitis. The severity of the nasal and ocular symptoms usually change in parallel. Physical findings include bilateral injection, erythema, and edema of the conjunctiva, accompanied by typical signs of nasal allergy. Skin tests or radioallergosorbent test (RAST) can be used to verify the diagnosis of allergy and to guide therapeutic decisions (Table 1).[1-3] Allergic conjunctivitis is examined in more detail in Chapter 5.

Allergic Rhinitis
Diagnostic features
Allergic rhinitis usually begins in childhood, and peak prevalence occurs in the 2nd and 3rd decades of life. Symptoms of allergic rhinitis include nasal congestion, rhinorrhea, nasal itching, and sneezing, occurring either seasonally or year-round. Associated physical findings include puffy eyes; swollen nasal mucosa that can be pale, bluish, or even red; nasal discharge that is usually clear and thin; serous effusion in the middle ear; and lymphoid aggregates on the soft palette and posterior pharynx. Skin tests or RAST can be used to confirm the diagnosis of respiratory allergy and to guide therapy (Table 2).[4-6] Allergic rhinitis is examined in more detail in Chapter 6.

Table 1: Differential Diagnosis of Allergic Conjunctivitis

Disorder	Frequency
Allergic rhinoconjunctivitis	Common
Atopic keratoconjunctivitis	Common
Contact dermatitis	Common
Giant papillary conjunctivitis	Common
Conjunctivitis sicca	Uncommon
Vernal conjunctivitis	Rare

Asthma

Diagnostic features

The diagnosis of asthma is based on the patient's medical history, physical examination, and objective measurements of pulmonary function. Cough, wheezing, and dyspnea that worsens in the early morning hours or with exercise are typical complaints. Moderate to severe asthma usually limits exercise tolerance, affects school or job performance, and wakens the patient at night. Wheezing of the chest is a main characteristic of asthma but is not always present because (1) airway obstruction in asthma is often erratic, so that examination of the chest during scheduled

Distinguishing features

Associated with allergic rhinitis
Positive skin tests or RAST
Bilateral conjunctival involvement

Usually associated with atopic dermatitis
elsewhere on the body
Bilateral prominent upper eyelid involvement

Associated with the use of a new eye drop or cosmetic
Distribution of rash corresponds to area where the
offending allergen was applied

Affects contact lens wearers
Papillary response on upper-lid conjunctiva
Symptoms fade if lenses are not worn

Decreased tearing
Associated with autoimmune disorders (Sjögren's
syndrome, mixed connective-tissue disease)

Affects children and young adults in tropical climates
Giant papillae on upper-lid conjunctiva

visits can be normal; (2) wheezing is a relatively insensitive sign of small-airway obstruction;[7] and (3) wheezing may be absent during severe exacerbations of asthma when airflow is severely limited. Other physical findings associated with asthma include the use of accessory muscles during tidal breathing (indicating severe airflow obstruction), a prolonged expiratory phase, and a barrel-chested appearance. Pulmonary function measurements that suggest asthma include reduction in forced expiratory volume in 1 second (FEV_1), peak expiratory flow (PEF), the ratio of FEV_1 to forced vital capacity (FEV_1/FVC ratio), and the midexpiratory flow rate (FEF_{25-75}).[8,9]

Table 2: Differential Diagnosis of Allergic Rhinitis

Disorder	Frequency
Allergic rhinitis	Common
Viral upper respiratory infection (URI)	Common
Bacterial sinusitis	Common
Foreign body	Common (young children)
NARES syndrome	Common
Vasomotor rhinitis	Common
Rhinitis medicamentosa	Common

Medication or drug side effects
  Antihypertensive drugs
  Cocaine abuse
  Birth control pills
	Common

Systemic conditions Pregnancy	Common
Hypothyroidism	Uncommon
Granulomatous diseases (Wegener's syndrome, sarcoidosis, infection)	Rare
Neoplasm	Rare
Mastocytosis	Rare

Distinguishing features

Chronic seasonal or perennial symptoms
Onset usually occurs in childhood
Positive skin tests or RAST

Self-limited illness lasting 5-10 days
Malaise or fever
Lymphadenopathy

Sinus radiographs abnormal
Halitosis
Purulent postnasal drip
Chronic cough: often follows a viral URI

Unilateral nasal discharge
Halitosis
Children <6 years of age

Eosinophilia of nasal secretions
Negative skin tests or RAST

Triggered by strong odors, tastes, or changes in climate
Negative skin tests or RAST

Use of topical vasoconstrictors for >5 days
Severe mucosal edema and erythema

Congestion temporally associated with beginning
a new medication

History and physical examination

Granulomatous lesions on rhinoscopy

Lesion seen on rhinoscopy
Mast cell infiltration of the skin, bone marrow, liver, spleen

Table 3: Differential Diagnosis of Asthma in Children

Disorder	Frequency
Asthma	Common
Bronchiolitis	Common
Chronic sinusitis	Common
Hyperventilation	Common
Laryngotracheomalacia	Common
Foreign body aspiration	Common
Vocal cord dysfunction	Common
Bronchopulmonary dysplasia	Uncommon
Gastroesophageal reflux with recurrent aspiration	Uncommon
Cystic fibrosis	Uncommon
Allergic bronchopulmonary aspergillosis	Rare

Congenital anatomic airway abnormality
    Vascular ring
    Laryngeal web
	Rare

Distinguishing features

Variable cough, wheeze, dyspnea
Worse at night and after exercise
Pulmonary function tests—reversible airway obstruction
Often associated with other atopic diseases
Symptoms relieved by β-agonist administration
Age < 2 years
Associated with respiratory syncytial virus or
parainfluenza infection
Chronic cough and nasal congestion
Abnormal sinus radiographs but normal pulmonary function
Triggered by anxiety or exercise
Normal pulmonary function tests, no hypoxia
Tingling or numbness of extremities
Rapid resolution of symptoms with calming
Stridor
Early onset of symptoms
No response to bronchodilator
Sudden onset of symptoms
Coughing or choking while eating
Abnormal expiratory chest radiograph (air trapping)
Bronchoscopy is the definitive study
Pulmonary function tests—decreased inspiratory flow
Hoarseness, stridor
Symptoms do not respond to asthma therapy
Chronic airway disease with exacerbations
History of premature delivery and respiratory support
Nocturnal symptoms common
Vomiting or cough when recumbent
Barium swallow abnormal
Abnormal sweat test and abnormal chest radiograph
Poor growth, fat malabsorption
Migratory infiltrates on chest radiograph
Positive skin test for *Aspergillus* (often with serum precipitins)
Elevated total IgE
Early onset of stridor, no response to bronchodilator
Airway compromised on chest radiograph or with barium swallow
Bronchoscopy

Table 4: Differential Diagnosis of Asthma in Adults

Disorder	Frequency
Asthma	Common
Chronic obstructive pulmonary disease	Common
Cardiac asthma	Common
Gastroesophageal reflux with recurrent aspiration	Common
Hyperventilation	Common
Vocal cord dysfunction	Common
Pulmonary embolism	Common
Hypersensitivity pneumonitis	Uncommon
Drug-induced cough	Uncommon

Distinguishing features

Variable cough, wheeze, dyspnea
Onset usually in childhood
Worse at night and with exercise
Pulmonary function tests—reversible airway obstruction
Often associated with other atopic diseases
Symptoms relieved by β-agonist administration

Progressive small airway obstruction
Poor response to bronchodilator
History of tobacco smoking

Physical signs of cardiac dysfunction
Chest radiograph—cardiomegaly
Abnormal echocardiogram

Nocturnal symptoms common
Vomiting or heartburn
Barium swallow

Triggered by anxiety or exercise
Normal pulmonary function tests, no hypoxia
Tingling or numbness of extremities
Rapid resolution of symptoms with calming

Hoarseness, stridor
Pulmonary function tests—limited inspiratory flow
Poor response to asthma therapy

Tachypnea, tachycardia
Hypoxia
Chest pain
Pulmonary function tests—restricted lung volume
Abnormal ventilation/perfusion scan

Occupational or recreational exposure to molds,
organic dusts, or chemical solvents
Antigen-specific, precipitating antibodies in serum
Pulmonary function tests—restricted lung volumes

Angiotensin-converting enzyme inhibitors

(continued on next page)

Table 4: Differential Diagnosis of Asthma in Adults (continued)

Disorder	Frequency
Fixed large-airway obstruction Vocal cord paralysis Tracheal stenosis Glottic web Foreign body Neoplasms	Uncommon
Allergic bronchopulmonary aspergillosis	Rare
Pulmonary infiltrates with eosinophilia syndromes	Rare
α_1-antitrypsin deficiency	Rare

A key feature of asthma is the demonstration of reversible airway obstruction. Reversibility is documented by performing pulmonary function tests (PEF or FEV_1) before and then 15 minutes after administration of a short-acting inhaled β-adrenergic agonist or by performing pulmonary function tests before and after a 2-week to 3-week course of oral or inhaled corticosteroid. An increase in PEF or FEV_1 of more than 12% from baseline values strongly supports the diagnosis of asthma[10] (Tables 3 and 4).[6,8,9,11-13] More information on asthma and its management is provided in Chapters 7 and 8.

Atopic Dermatitis
Diagnostic features
Atopic dermatitis is a chronic skin disorder characterized by pruritus, dry skin, and excoriation. It can be local-

Distinguishing features

Stridor
Pulmonary function tests—decreased inspiratory and expiratory flow
No bronchodilator response
Abnormal chest radiograph (neoplasm)
Bronchoscopy

Migratory infiltrates on chest radiograph
Positive skin test for *Aspergillus*
Elevated total IgE
Aspergillus precipitins in serum

Pulmonary infiltrates
Peripheral blood eosinophilia

Emphysema
Low or undetectable serum α_1-antitrypsin
α_1-antitrypsin phenotype abnormal

ized to a few patches or involve large portions of the body. Atopic dermatitis usually begins early in life, typically in the second half of the first year. The pattern of distribution of atopic dermatitis lesions changes with age. Affected areas in infants include the cheeks, trunk, and extensor surfaces of the extremities. During childhood and adolescence, the distribution shifts to involve the neck and flexural areas of the extremities.

Early lesions of atopic dermatitis are red and dry, with small papules, mild scaling, and areas of excoriation. Skin infections are common, and appear as moist and oozing lesions, or as sudden onset of intense erythema of the affected skin. Chronically affected areas show accentuated skin lines and thickening of the skin (lichenification) and postinflammatory pigmentation abnormalities. Pruritus is universally present, and scratching is a major factor in the pathogenesis

Table 5: Differential Diagnosis of Atopic Dermatitis

Disorder	Frequency
Atopic dermatitis	Common
Seborrheic dermatitis	Common
Scabies	Common
Contact dermatitis	Common
Nummular dermatitis	Common
Drug eruption	Common
Immune deficiency	
Wiskott-Aldrich syndrome	Rare
Severe combined immunodeficiency	Rare
Hyperimmunoglobulinemia E syndrome	Rare

of the acute and chronic skin lesions (Table 5).[14,15] Atopic and contact dermatitis are examined in Chapter 10.

Food Allergy
Diagnostic features

Food-induced allergic reactions usually begin soon after the ingestion of the offending food, often within minutes

Distinguishing features

Pruritus
Characteristic distribution:
- Infants—cheeks, trunk, and extensor surfaces
- Children and adults—flexor surfaces

Associated with other atopic diseases
Nonpruritic
Greasy scale on scalp, nasal folds, behind ears
Onset soon after birth
Intertriginous papules
Mites visualized in scraping of lesions
Contagious
Onset corresponds with use of new medicine or skin cream
Distribution of rash corresponds to area of contact
with the offending allergen
Lesions limited to small, round, scaly plaques
Coincides with beginning a new oral or
parenteral medication
Thrombocytopenia
Chronic diarrhea
Recurrent infections
Lymphopenia
Chronic diarrhea and recurrent infections
Staphylococcal abscesses and pneumonitis
Very high total serum IgE (but IgE levels overlap
with those of atopic dermatitis)

and nearly always within 2 hours. The gastrointestinal tract and the skin are the most commonly affected organ systems. Reactions range in severity from flushing or mild itching of the mouth to wheezing, upper airway obstruction, and cardiovascular collapse (see Anaphylaxis, below). Abdominal pain, nausea, vomiting, and diarrhea are gastrointestinal symptoms commonly associated with food aller-

31

Table 6: Differential Diagnosis of Food Allergy

Disorder	Frequency
Food allergy	Common
Toxic contamination of food • Bacterial toxins • Scombroid fish poisoning	Common
Impaired food absorption • Lactase deficiency (milk) • Fructose overload (fruit juice) • Sorbitol (sugarless gum or candy)	Common
Pharmacologic properties of food • Coffee (caffeine) • Aged cheese (tyramine)	Common
Idiosyncratic responses • Alcohol-flushing • Chinese restaurant syndrome	Common
Psychosomatic reactions	Uncommon
Allergy to food dyes or preservatives	Uncommon
Inflammatory bowel disease	Uncommon
Anorexia nervosa/bulimia	Uncommon
Inborn errors of metabolism • Sucrase-isomaltase deficiency • Phenylketonuria • Many others	Rare

Distinguishing features

Typical organ systems involved
Temporally associated with causative food
Reproducible each time offending food is eaten
Associated with other atopic diseases
Positive skin tests or RAST in most cases

Affects a large percentage of people ingesting the food
Includes toxins from *S aureus, Shigella, E coli*
Elevated histamine levels from breakdown of
histidine in the meat of deep-sea fish

Bloating, diarrhea, and intestinal gas
Small amounts are usually tolerated but symptoms
develop if absorption capacity is exceeded

Symptoms are produced only when large quantities of
the food are ingested

Reproducible, but mechanisms are unknown

Not reproducible with double-blind, placebo-
controlled food challenges

Verify with double-blind, placebo-controlled food
challenge

Abnormal abdominal radiographs
Elevated erythrocyte sedimentation rate
Intolerance for a broad range of foods

Distorted body image
Intolerance for a broad range of foods

Failure to thrive
Vomiting, diarrhea
Seizures

Table 7: Differential Diagnosis of Anaphylaxis

Disorder	Frequency
Anaphylaxis	Common
Vasovagal reactions	Common
Asthma	Common
Arrhythmia, myocardial infarction	Common
Food aspiration	Common
Serum sickness	Common
Idiopathic urticaria	Common
Pulmonary embolus	Uncommon
Sepsis	Uncommon
Flushing syndrome	
• Mastocytosis	Rare
• Carcinoid tumor	Rare
Scombroid fish poisoning	Rare

gy. Multiple vague complaints, such as lethargy and headache, without signs or symptoms of hypersensitivity, are unlikely to be from food allergy.[16]

Testing for food-specific IgE either by prick skin testing or RAST can provide data to support or disprove the possi-

Distinguishing features

Typical organ systems involved (skin, respiratory, cardiovascular, gastrointestinal tract)
Usually abrupt onset
Hypotension and tachycardia
Elevated serum tryptase (retrospectively)

Triggered by pain or anxiety
Hypotension and bradycardia
Pallor, diaphoresis
Rapid recovery when feet are elevated

No skin manifestations or hypotension

Abnormal electrocardiogram
Findings limited to cardiovascular compromise

Abrupt onset of coughing and choking during a meal

Gradual onset of rash, fever, arthritis
Occurs 7-21 days after starting a new medication

Findings limited to the skin

Tachypnea and tachycardia
Absence of wheezing and urticaria

Fever, progressive illness

Mast cell infiltration of the skin, bone marrow, liver, spleen
Elevated urine 5-hydroxyindoleacetic acid

Flushing, sometimes wheezing, after eating deep-sea fish (due to histamine in the meat)

bility of food allergy, but both tests have a low positive predictive value. Double-blind, placebo-controlled food challenge is the best method for confirming the diagnosis of food allergy (Table 6).[17-19] More information on food allergy is provided in Chapter 11.

Anaphylaxis
Diagnostic features

Anaphylaxis is usually a clinical diagnosis. In most cases, there is a clear history of a sudden and sometimes catastrophic reaction that closely follows the administration of an inciting agent, but in some cases, no cause can be identified. Signs and symptoms of anaphylaxis include (1) urticaria, angioedema, and flushing; (2) rhinorrhea, bronchospasm, hoarseness, and laryngeal edema; (3) capillary leakage, diminished cardiac output, tachycardia, and hypotension; (4) nausea, vomiting, abdominal pain, and diarrhea; and (5) loss of consciousness. Laboratory evaluation is usually not helpful during the acute reaction; however, finding an increase in serum tryptase, a mast-cell mediator, can retrospectively confirm the diagnosis of anaphylaxis (Table 7).[20-22] Anaphylaxis is examined in more detail in Chapter 14.

References

1. Weiss A, Brinser JH, Nazar-Stewart V: Acute conjunctivitis in childhood. *J Pediatr* 1993;122:10-14.

2. Trocme SD, Raizman MB, Bartley GB: Medical therapy for ocular allergy. *Mayo Clin Proc* 1992;67:557-565.

3. Bielory L: Allergic and immunologic disorders of the eye. Part II: ocular allergy. *J Allergy Clin Immunol* 2000;106:1019-1032.

4. Naclerio RM: Allergic rhinitis. *N Engl J Med* 1991;325: 860-869.

5. Jacobs RL, Freedman PM, Boswell RN: Nonallergic rhinitis with eosinophilia (NARES syndrome). Clinical and immunologic presentation. *J Allergy Clin Immunol* 1981;67:253-262.

6. Busse WW, Holgate ST, eds: *Asthma and Rhinitis*. Oxford, Blackwell Scientific Publications, 2000.

7. Shim CS, Williams MH Jr: Relationship of wheezing to the severity of obstruction in asthma. *Arch Intern Med* 1983;143: 890-892.

8. National Asthma Education Program and Prevention, National Heart, Lung, and Blood Institute, National Institutes of Health: Expert Panel Report II: *Guidelines for the Diagnosis and Management of Asthma*. Bethesda, US Department of Health and Human Services, 1997.

9. National Asthma Education Program: *Practical guide for the diagnosis and management of asthma.* Bethesda, US Department of Health and Human Services, 1997.

10. American Thoracic Society: Lung function testing: selection of reference values and interpretative strategies. *Am Rev Respir Dis* 1991;144:1202-1218.

11. Landau LI: Bronchiolitis and asthma: are they related? *Thorax* 1994;49:293-296.

12. Gern JE, Schroth MK, Lemanske RF Jr: Childhood asthma. Older children and adolescents. *Clin Chest Med* 1995;16:657-670.

13. American Thoracic Society: Standards for the diagnosis and care of patients with chronic obstructive pulmonary disease (COPD) and asthma. *Am Rev Respir Dis* 1987;136:225-244.

14. Przybilla B, Eberlein-Konig B, Rueff F: Practical management of atopic eczema. *Lancet* 1994;343:1342-1346.

15. Boguniewicz M, Leung DY: Atopic dermatitis. In: Middleton E Jr, Reed CE, Ellis EF, et al, eds. *Allergy: Principles and Practice.* St. Louis, Mosby-Year Book, 1998, pp 1123-1134.

16. Pearson DJ, Rix KJ, Bentley SJ: Food allergy: how much in the mind? A clinical and psychiatric study of suspected food hypersensitivity. *Lancet* 1983;1:1259-1261.

17. Sampson HA: Food allergy. *JAMA* 1997;278:1888-1894.

18. Anderson JA: Food allergy, science and reason. *N Engl Reg Allergy Proc* 1986;7:501-503.

19. Metcalfe DD, Sampson HA, Simon RA: *Food Allergy.* Boston, Blackwell Scientific Publications, 1997.

20. Bochner BS, Lichtenstein LM: Anaphylaxis. *N Engl J Med* 1991;324:1785-1790.

21. Joint Task Force on Practice Parameters, American Academy of Allergy, Asthma and Immunology, American College of Allergy, Asthma and Immunology, and the Joint Council of Allergy, Asthma and Immunology: The diagnosis and management of anaphylaxis. *J Allergy Clin Immunol* 1998;101:S466-S528.

22. Winbery SL, Lieberman PL: Anaphylaxis. In: Virant SL, ed: *Systemic Reactions.* Philadelphia, WB Saunders, 1995, pp 447-475.

3

Pathogenesis of Allergies and Asthma

Overview of Allergic Mechanisms

Allergy and hypersensitivity are terms that are used interchangeably to describe an adverse clinical reaction to a foreign substance caused by an immunologic mechanism. Gell and Coombs originally proposed several different mechanisms for immunologic hypersensitivity, and Shearer and Huston[1] have modified the classification system to accommodate more recent discoveries (Table 1). Common respiratory, food, and stinging insect allergies and some drug reactions are mediated by mast cells. These are known as type I hypersensitivity reactions, or *immediate* hypersensitivity. Mast cells can be triggered via either immunoglobulin E (IgE)-dependent or IgE-independent (anaphylactoid) pathways. Several drugs, such as codeine and radiocontrast media, can precipitate anaphylactoid reactions by inducing degranulation of mast cells without binding to IgE.[2] Aspirin and other nonsteroidal anti-inflammatory drugs (NSAIDs) can produce similar reactions but do so through a distinct mechanism. NSAIDs inhibit the enzyme prostaglandin synthase (cyclooxygenase) and thereby block the synthesis of prostaglandins from arachidonic acid. In aspirin-sensitive individuals, however, the reduction in prostaglandin synthesis is accompanied by increased production of the other major derivatives of arachidonic acid, the leuko-

Table 1: Classification of Hypersensitivity Reactions*

Type I	Mast cell mediated a) IgE-dependent (anaphylactic) b) IgE-independent (anaphylactoid)
Type II	Antibody-mediated (non-IgE)
Type III	Immune complex
Type IV	Cell mediated

*Modified from Shearer and Huston,[1] used with permission.

trienes.[3] Overproduction of leukotrienes, which are potent bronchoconstrictors and vasodilators, may produce severe allergic symptoms.

Type II hypersensitivity reactions occur when antibodies (other than IgE) bind to the surface of cells or to extracellular tissues, leading to activation of complement and phagocytic cells. Penicillin can produce type II reactions by binding to the surface of red blood cells, creating a *neoantigen* that may be recognized by circulating antibodies. Binding of the antibody to the surface of the red cell leads to activation of complement and cell lysis.[4]

Type III reactions occur when antibodies bind to circulating antigens and form immune complexes, which are also potent activators of complement. This type of reaction was recognized early this century by Clemens von Pirquet, who observed that patients receiving horse serum as treatment for diphtheria developed skin rash, arthritis, and fever. Similar reactions have recently been observed in patients receiving antithymocyte globulin as treatment for bone marrow failure.[5]

Finally, type IV reactions, also known as delayed-type hypersensitivity reactions, are mediated by T lymphocytes or natural killer cells. Examples include skin rashes that occur 1 to 2 days after contact with poison ivy, nickel, or other skin sensitizers in susceptible individuals. Type IV reactions require a sensitization phase, during which the antigen is processed by antigen-presenting cells that then activate CD4+ T cells.[6] Within 48 hours of reexposure, both antigen-specific and antigen-nonspecific T cells home to the area of exposure. Cytokines secreted by activated T cells recruit additional mononuclear cells into the area and potentiate the inflammatory functions of cells in the affected tissue.

These different types of reactions are not mutually exclusive, and an allergen can produce more than one type of reaction even in a single individual. For example, reactions to latex gloves may progress over time from contact dermatitis to contact urticaria to anaphylaxis.[7] Of course, many types of adverse reactions to foreign substances do not involve immunologic mechanisms. Examples include irritant reactions (nasal irritation after exposure to tobacco smoke), pharmacologic effects of a substance (local swelling after a bee sting), metabolic deficiencies (diarrhea secondary to lactase deficiency), and idiosyncratic reactions for which no mechanism has been identified. In most cases, these reactions may be distinguished from allergy by careful evaluation of the history and physical findings.

Allergens

Allergens are substances that lead to sensitization (ie, production of allergen-specific IgE) followed by induction of clinical symptoms of allergy upon reexposure. Most allergens are medium-sized proteins that bind to specific IgE molecules on the surface of mast cells and basophils, triggering the release of a cascade of inflammatory mediators. Low-molecular-weight substances (haptens) such as penicillin metabolites are too small to cross-link IgE on their own, but they may serve as allergens after binding to carrier proteins such as albumin.

Allergens come from a wide variety of sources, and exposure may occur by inhalation, ingestion, or injection (Table 2). Respiratory allergens may be classified as either perennial

Table 2: Common Allergens

Inhaled	Ingested	Injected

• Pollens
  - Trees
  - Grasses
  - Weeds
• Molds
  - *Alternaria*
  - *Aspergillus*
• Arthropods
  - House
    dust mite
  - Cockroach
• Animal
  proteins
  - Cat
  - Rodents
  - Dog
• Latex
	• Foods
	  - Egg
	  - Milk
	  - Soy
	  - Peanut
	  - Tree nuts
	  - Fish
	• Medications
	  - Penicillin
	  - Cephalo-
	    sporins
	  - Sulfonamide
	  - Erythromycin
	  - Codeine
		• Insect venom
		  - Yellow
		    jacket
		  - Bee
		  - Wasp
		  - Fire ant
		• Medications
		  - Penicillin
		  - Cephalo-
		    sporins
		  - Morphine*
		• Intravenous
		  contrast dye*

*Substances that provoke allergic reactions through IgE-independent mechanisms

(year-round) or seasonal, depending on their patterns of exposure. Common perennial allergens include proteins from house dust mites, pets, cockroaches, rodents, and indoor molds. Seasonal allergens include pollens from trees, grasses, and weeds, in addition to outdoor molds such as *Alternaria*. Extracts prepared from these allergens have long been used in the diagnosis and treatment of allergy and naturally contain many proteins and other soluble substances. The past 2 decades have witnessed a significant effort to identify the specific proteins responsible for producing allergic symptoms and to develop standardized extracts containing defined amounts of allergenic protein.[8]

The major allergenic proteins for house dust mite, cat, ragweed, and many other major allergens have been identified, and in some instances, the genes have been cloned and sequenced. These allergenic extracts are now being standardized according to allergen content and skin test reactivity, and this has improved the potency, reliability, efficacy, and safety of these preparations.

Allergen Sensitization

Allergen sensitization refers to a process in which a foreign protein interacts with the immune system, leading to the production of allergen-specific IgE. Once an individual becomes sensitized, additional contacts with the allergen may produce signs and symptoms of allergy. Several factors determine the likelihood of sensitization to a particular antigen. Sensitization most readily occurs with repetitive exposure to an allergen via the mucous membranes, skin, or gastrointestinal tract. It is less common after parenteral exposure. High doses of allergen are also more likely to produce sensitization.[9] Host factors that influence sensitization rates include age (peak incidence in the 2nd decade of life) and genetic factors. Although the genetics of allergy are far from clear, detailed analyses of allergic families have revealed that certain class II major compatibility loci are linked to the production of allergen-specific IgE.[10] In contrast, total serum IgE levels show linkage to several markers on chromosome 5, including the gene for interleukin-4 (IL-4), a cytokine that is required for IgE production.[11]

Regulation of IgE Synthesis

Production of allergen-specific IgE is prerequisite to the development of type I allergic reactions. Thus, defining the regulation of this process is important in efforts to find effective treatments and perhaps even a cure for allergy. Produc-

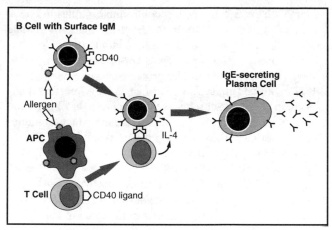

Figure 1: Regulation of IgE synthesis. A protein allergen activates a resting B cell by binding to surface IgM and activates T cells after first being processed by an antigen-presenting cell (APC). For IgE synthesis to occur, the T cell must furnish two signals by binding to CD40 on the B cell and secreting interleukin-4. These stimuli allow for isotype switching from IgM to IgE, followed by differentiation of the B cell into an IgE-secreting plasma cell.

tion of IgE requires a cooperative effort of CD4+ T cells ('helper T cells') and B cells (Figure 1). After maturing in the bone marrow, B cells have IgM or IgD immunoglobulin on their cell membrane (surface immunoglobulin). The immunoglobulin produced by each B cell has a unique structure in the antigen-binding region (variable portion of the Fab region). As a result, each B cell can bind a unique antigen, such as house dust mite protein. For a B cell to become activated to produce the secreted form of immunoglobulin, there must be at least two signals.[12] One signal occurs when the surface immunoglobulin on the B cell binds to an antigen. The second signal is provided by T helper cells that are activated by the same antigen. The activated T cells make contact with the B cell, and a second signal is transmitted via the CD40 surface protein on the B cell. These two signals cause the B cell to further differentiate into immunoglobulin-secreting plasma cells. The signals also cause an *isotype shift* in the type of immunoglobulin produced, so that IgG, IgA, or IgE is produced instead of IgM or IgD. A major breakthrough in allergy research was the discovery that T cells and other cells secrete cytokines that determine which immunoglobulin isotype will be produced. For example, IL-4 or interleukin-13 (IL-13) is necessary for the switch from IgM to IgE secretion, while interferon-γ (IFN-γ) favors the production of IgG. Identification of the mechanism for the production of allergen-specific IgE has led to the development of new experimental approaches to controlling allergies and asthma.

Pathogenesis of Type I Hypersensitivity Reactions

There has been an explosion of information about the pathogenesis of allergy in the past decade. Perhaps the most important concept that has come out of recent discoveries is that symptoms of respiratory allergy are directly related to an allergen-driven chronic inflammation of the respiratory mucosa. Whether it is present in the eye, nose, or small airways of the lung, allergic inflammation acts on local structures such as smooth muscle, epithelial cells, and nerves to produce an increased sensitivity of the affected tissue to specific allergens (eg, pollen, house dust mite) and irritants (eg, tobacco smoke, cold air). This heightened sensitivity to allergic as well as nonspecific stimuli is called *hyperresponsiveness*.[13] Bronchial hyperresponsiveness can be measured by performing an inhalational challenge using a nonspecific stimulus such as methacholine, histamine, or cold air and then measuring the degree of bronchoconstriction using spirometry.[14] This concept has been valuable in understanding the relationship between inflammation and clinical symptoms and as a diagnostic tool in patients with symptoms that suggest asthma.

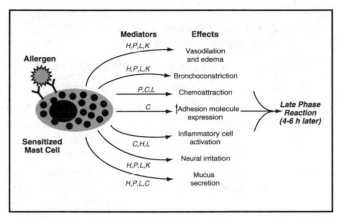

Figure 2: Effects of allergen-induced release of mast cell mediators. H = histamine; P = prostaglandin D_2; L = leukotrienes; K = kinins; C = cytokines.

Although many cells and mediators participate in allergy pathogenesis, it is clear that a few are key in this process. Allergens that reach the target tissue bind to allergen-specific IgE on the surface of mast cells, basophils, and other cells bearing IgE receptors. When IgE molecules are cross-linked by an allergen, the mast cell releases preformed mediators present in intracellular granules and begins to synthesize and secrete additional mediators and cytokines (Figure 2). Alternately, mast cells may be triggered directly by low-molecular-weight substances such as codeine or intravenous contrast material. Mediators contained in granules, such as histamine, produce vasodilation and increase capillary leakage within minutes, and newly synthesized leukotrienes and prostaglandins exacerbate local inflammation and attract new inflammatory cells such as eosinophils, basophils, and activated T cells into the area.[15]

Cytokines produced by mast cells, T cells, and other inflammatory cells have many proinflammatory effects, including enhancement of endothelial cell adhesion molecule

Table 3: Cytokines Implicated in Allergic Inflammation

Cytokine	Cell Sources	Pertinent Effects
Eotaxin	Mononuclear cells, epithelial cells	• Eosinophil chemoattractant
IL-3	T cells	• Mast cell and basophil growth factor
IL-4	T cells, basophils	• IgE synthesis • Recruits eosinophils to site via effects on adhesion molecule VCAM-1
IL-5	T cells, mast cells	• Eosinophil growth factor • Potent eosinophil activator
GM-CSF	T cells, epithelial and endothelial cells, eosinophils	• Granulocyte growth factor • Eosinophil activator
RANTES	Platelets, epithelial cells, macrophages	• Eosinophil chemoattractant
TNF-α	Macrophages, mast cells	• ↑Adhesion molecule expression • ↑Capillary permeability • ↑Mucus secretion

Table 4: Cells Involved in Chronic Allergic Inflammation

Cell	Mediators	Comments
Basophil, mast cell	Histamine, LTB_4, C_4, cytokines (IL-4, TNF)	Has high-affinity IgE receptors on surface and is triggered by allergen
Dendritic cell	Cytokines (IL-1, TNF)	Avid antigen-presenting cell and T-cell activator
Eosinophil	Cationic granular proteins, superoxide, LTC_4, cytokines (GM-CSF)	Granule proteins arc toxic to epithelial cells, irritating to neurons
Macrophage	Superoxide, nitric oxide, PGE_2, LTB_4, cytokines (IL-1, TNF, GM-CSF)	Macrophages have considerable inflammatory capabilities and can activate other cells via antigen presentation or cytokine secretion
T cell	Cytokines (IL-3, IL-4, IL-5, GM-CSF)	Cytokines secreted by allergen-specific T cells are potent activators of eosinophils and IgE production

expression leading to additional cell recruitment[16] and augmentation of inflammatory cell function (Table 3). These inflammatory cells, particularly eosinophils, secrete additional mediators and cytokines that damage epithelial cells, stimulate mucus secretion and neurogenic inflammation, and promote vascular leakage and tissue edema (Table 4).[17]

In the respiratory tract, each of these factors contributes to nasal and lower-airway obstruction, leading directly to clinical symptoms. With continued allergen exposure, inflammation may progress to structural changes in the airway, such as increased collagen deposition, hypertrophy of airway smooth muscle, and vascular hyperplasia. These changes, known as airway remodeling, are likely to contribute to long-term, perhaps irreversible, deterioration in lung function.[18]

Summary

Because many factors contribute to the pathogenesis of allergy and asthma, interventions at multiple levels may be required to control these disorders. Defining allergic mechanisms has enabled the development of therapies that affect one or more specific mediators or effector cells described in this review. A clear understanding of the pathogenesis of allergy will enable clinicians to most effectively use current and future generations of antiallergic therapies.

References

1. Shearer WT, Huston DP: The immune system. In: Middleton E Jr, Reed CE, Ellis EF, et al, eds. *Allergy: Principles and Practice*. St. Louis, Mosby-Year Book, 1993, pp 3-21.

2. VanArsdel PP Jr: Pseudoallergic drug reactions. *Immunol Allergy Clin North Am* 1991;11:635-644.

3. Israel E, Fischer AR, Rosenberg MA, et al: The pivotal role of 5-lipoxygenase products in the reaction of aspirin-sensitive asthmatics to aspirin. *Am Rev Respir Dis* 1993;148:1447-1451.

4. Dove AF, Thomas DJ, Aronstam A, et al: Haemolytic anaemia due to penicillin. *Br Med J* 1975;3:684.

5. Lawley TJ, Bielory L, Gascon P, et al: A prospective clinical and immunologic analysis of patients with serum sickness. *N Engl J Med* 1984;311:1407-1413.

6. Wood GS, Volterra AS, Abel EA, et al: Allergic contact dermatitis: novel immunohistologic features. *J Invest Dermatol* 1986;87:688-693.

7. Ownby DR: Manifestations of latex allergy. *Immunol Allergy Clin North Am* 1995;15:31-43.

8. Ipsen H, Larsen JN, Neimeijer NR, et al: Allergenic extracts. In: Middleton E Jr, Reed CE, Ellis EF, et al, eds. *Allergy: Principles and Practice*. St. Louis, Mosby-Year Book, 1998, pp 404-416.

9. Bachmann MF, Rohrer UH, Steinhoff U, et al: T helper cell unresponsiveness: rapid induction in antigen-transgenic and reversion in non-transgenic mice. *Eur J Immunol* 1994;24:2966-2973.

10. Meyers DA, Freidhoff LR, Marsh DG: Predicting skin test sensitivity and total serum IgE levels in family members. *J Allergy Clin Immunol* 1986;77:608-615.

11. Barnes KC: Evidence for common genetic elements in allergic disease. *J Allergy Clin Immunol* 2000;106:S192-S200.

12. Vercelli D: Molecular regulation of the IgE immune response. *Clin Exp Allergy* 1995;25:43-45.

13. Colasurdo GN, Larsen GL: Airway hyperresponsiveness. In: Busse WW, Holgate ST, eds. *Asthma and Rhinitis*. Boston, Blackwell Scientific Publications, 1995, pp 1044-1056.

14. Townley RJ, Hopp RJ: Inhalation methods for the study of airway responsiveness. *J Allergy Clin Immunol* 1987;80:111-124.

15. Busse WW, Lemanske RF Jr: Asthma. *N Engl J Med* 2001; 344:350-362.

16. Montefort S, Holgate ST, Howarth PH: Leucocyte-endothelial adhesion molecules and their role in bronchial asthma and allergic rhinitis. *Eur Respir J* 1993;6:1044-1054.

17. Kay AB, Barata L, Meng Q, et al: Eosinophil and eosinophil-associated cytokines in allergic inflammation. *Int Arch Allergy Immunol* 1997;113:196-199.

18. Reed CE: The natural history of asthma in adults: the problem of irreversibility. *J Allergy Clin Immunol* 1999;103:539-547.

4

Testing for Allergy

B ecause seasonal allergies are often clinically obvious, they usually can be treated appropriately without skin testing or in vitro assays. In more ambiguous cases or in those involving perennial symptoms, testing for allergy provides information that helps to establish the correct diagnosis, to formulate measures that control exposure to environmental allergens, and to prescribe medication or immunotherapy. The detection of allergen-specific IgE is the most useful test in evaluating the possibility of immediate hypersensitivity,[1,2] although other tests can provide supportive information or be used to rule out other disorders in the differential diagnosis. This chapter reviews the indications, methods, and interpretation of skin and laboratory testing for allergy.

Laboratory Tests
Eosinophil count

Allergic individuals often have increased circulating eosinophils, and blood eosinophil counts correlate with disease severity in atopic dermatitis[3] and asthma.[4] However, because of large variations among individuals, the eosinophil count cannot be relied upon as a sensitive marker for either the presence or the severity of allergic disease in a particular individual.

Table 1: Indications to Test for Allergen-Specific IgE

Inhalant sensitivity
- Allergic rhinitis
- Asthma

Food sensitivity
- Severe atopic dermatitis (children)
- Food-induced respiratory symptoms
- Food-induced gastrointestinal symptoms
- Food-induced urticaria or anaphylaxis

Drug reactions
- Penicillin sensitivity
- Local anesthetic reactions

Stinging insect anaphylaxis

Latex hypersensitivity

Examining nasal secretions for eosinophils is sometimes useful in diagnosing allergic rhinitis in patients with chronic nasal symptoms.[5] During active allergic rhinitis, the nasal secretions may contain more than 25% eosinophils. However, nonallergic individuals with NARES (nonallergic rhinitis with eosinophilia syndrome) also have eosinophilia of the nasal secretions without respiratory allergies.[6] Many individuals with NARES have a good response to topical corticosteroids.

Total serum IgE

There is no doubt that the mean total serum immunoglobulin E (IgE) level of allergic patients is elevated; however, there is considerable overlap with total serum IgE levels of nonallergic individuals.[7] As a result, the total serum IgE

Table 2: Selection of Skin Tests Versus RAST

Skin tests	RAST
• Greater sensitivity	• Not affected by antihistamines
• Measure biologic response	• Not affected by skin disease
• Less expensive	• No risk of anaphylaxis
• Rapid results	• Widely available

level is not very useful in evaluating individuals with suspected allergy.[2,7] The preferred diagnostic test for allergy is the detection of allergen-specific IgE antibodies using an appropriate panel of allergen skin tests or radioallergosorbent test (RAST).

Detection of allergen-specific IgE

Allergen-specific IgE can be measured using immediate hypersensitivity skin tests or in vitro methods, such as the RAST or analogs thereof. Indications for skin testing or RAST include the clinical suspicion of respiratory allergy (rhinoconjunctivitis or asthma) or allergy to foods, stinging insects, or latex (Table 1).

The decision to use skin tests or RAST to detect allergen-specific IgE is based largely on availability and expertise, but each technique has advantages and disadvantages that affect its clinical utility (Table 2). Because the reliability of allergy test results strongly depends on technical factors, health-care providers should refer to qualified allergists or laboratories who use strict quality control measures. Skin testing is somewhat more sensitive and specific,[2] yields information quickly, is relatively inexpensive, and is the preferred method for detecting IgE-mediated reactions to medications such as penicillin.[8]

Table 3: Contraindications to Allergen Skin Testing

Absolute
- Patient is on β-blocker therapy
- Pregnancy
- Generalized skin disease

Relative
- History of severe anaphylaxis
- Dermatographism
- Use of H_1 antihistamines, which inhibit the skin-test response for variable periods:
  - Hydroxyzine, cetirizine, loratadine—3-10 days
  - Fexofenadine—2 days
  - Other antihistamines—1-3 days
  - Tricyclic antidepressants—5 days

Contraindications to skin testing (Table 3) include the use of β-blockers such as propranolol (Inderal®) or metoprolol (Lopressor®, Toprol-XL®). If anaphylaxis occurs in a patient taking β-blockers, resuscitative efforts with epinephrine (Ana-Kit®, Epipen®, Epipen® Jr.) may be unsuccessful, so there is an increased risk for a fatal reaction.[9] Pregnancy is also a contraindication to skin testing. Although the risk of anaphylaxis induced by skin testing is low, such a reaction during pregnancy could harm the fetus.[10] Skin tests are not useful in patients with extensive skin disease or in those receiving antihistamines because these factors may obscure wheal and flare responses.

RAST and RAST analogs are useful when skin tests are contraindicated or cannot be interpreted because of concurrent skin disorders such as severe atopic dermatitis or dermatographism, or when it is not desirable to stop antihistamine therapy (Table 2). Disadvantages of RAST include the relatively high cost, decreased sensitivity and specificity compared to skin tests, and a turnaround time of several days or more.

Methods

Skin testing can be performed using either the prick or the intradermal technique.[11,12] Prick skin tests are simple, rapid, relatively painless, and commonly used as screening tests. Prick skin tests are generally considered to be more specific than intradermal tests because there are fewer false-positive reactions. Also, adverse reactions are more common with intradermal testing because of the larger dose of antigen administered; therefore, prick skin testing should be done first to minimize the risk of systemic allergic reactions. Prick skin tests are also preferred in testing for food allergy because of the lower incidence of false-positive tests compared to intradermal testing. The extracts used in prick skin testing are usually 1:10 to 1:20 weight per volume extracts in 50% glycerine, and every effort should be made to use standardized extracts from reputable sources. Control solutions include histamine (1 mg/mL for prick testing) and the diluent used to prepare the extract. After application of a drop of extract, the skin is pricked with a bifurcated needle, blood lancet, or commercially available multitest device.[13] Intradermal testing involves the intradermal injection of 0.03 mL to 0.05 mL of diluted (1:100-1:1000) extract. The test results (size of wheal and flare) of either mode of testing are read 10 to 15 minutes later.

Skin test results depend on a number of factors besides the presence of IgE, such as mast cell degranulation and the responsiveness of the skin to inflammatory mediators such as histamine. Therefore, skin testing provides a more informative evaluation of the effect of the allergic reac-

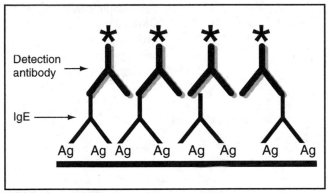

Figure 1: Radioallergosorbent test. Antigen (Ag) is bound to a solid support such as nitrocellulose, paper disks, or beads. Test serum is then incubated with the solid-phase antigen, and antigen-specific antibody (if present) binds to antigen. To detect allergen-specific IgE, a labeled (*) detection antibody specific for IgE is added, and quantitative measurements are performed in either a scintillation counter (radioactivity) or an ELISA plate reader (enzyme detection system).

tion than simply measuring specific IgE antibodies in serum. However, antihistamines may suppress skin-test responses for variable periods of time (Table 3).[14] Tricyclic antidepressants can also blunt the skin test response for up to 5 days.

The RAST and RAST analogs are in vitro tests designed to detect allergen-specific IgE antibodies in serum.[15] The test involves the coupling or absorption of an allergenic protein onto a solid-phase support such as microcrystalline cellulose, paper disks, sepharose beads, or nitrocellulose (Figure 1). Human serum is incubated with the solid-phase antigen, and the allergen-specific IgE antibodies are detected by the addition of antihuman IgE antibodies labeled with radioactive iodine or an enzyme.

Table 4: Selection of Tests for Allergen-Specific IgE

Indoor

- House dust mite
- Molds
  - *Aspergillus*
  - *Penicillium*
  - *Cladosporium*
- Pets and pests
  - Cat
  - Dog
  - Mouse
  - Cockroach

Selection of Specific Allergens for Testing

The number of skin tests or RAST performed should not be excessive because the information gained from a few tests chosen based on the pattern of symptoms and history of exposure is more relevant than information derived from a large number of tests selected as a 'panel' (Table 4). When selecting allergens for testing, either by in vivo or in vitro methods, clinicians should consider several factors.[16] First, what is the likelihood that identification of these allergens will improve the quality of the patient's care, either by avoidance measures or by intervention with medications or immunotherapy? Second, the specific allergens used in the testing should be chosen according to the nature of the allergens found in the patient's locale. Pollens from trees, grasses, and weeds vary in different parts of the United States. Thus, a knowledge of the botany of the area where the patient lives will be of use in determining which materials to choose for testing and whether treatment with immunotherapy is appropriate. Third, the age of the patient should influence allergen selection. For example, children may develop allergies to foods in the first few months of age but are rarely allergic to indoor allergens before the age of 1 to 2 years, or to pollens before 4 to 5 years of age.[17] Finally, the availabili-

Outdoor

Season	Predominant allergens
Spring	Trees
Summer	Grasses, molds (late)
Fall	Molds (*Alternaria*), weeds

ty of standardized materials for skin testing or RAST should be considered. The use of poorly characterized reagents or inappropriate allergens such as butterfly, tobacco smoke, or facial tissue extracts should be avoided.

Indoor Allergens

Because house dust mite sensitivity is a major cause of allergic respiratory disease,[18] testing for house dust mites is essential. The two chief species of house dust mite in the United States are *Dermatophagoides pteronyssinus* and *D farinae*, and standardized extracts are available for testing.

Pet proteins are another major source of indoor allergens and have been linked to allergic rhinitis and asthma.[18] The main allergen responsible for cat allergy is the protein *Fel d 1*, which is found in cat dander and cat saliva. The chief allergens responsible for dog allergy are less well characterized than cat antigens and may be specific for a particular breed.[19] Rodents such as rabbits, hamsters, and gerbils are also highly allergenic. The major rodent allergens are excreted in the urine.[20]

Molds such as *Aspergillus* and *Penicillium* are also indoor allergens.[21] These grow best on moist areas such as basements, bathroom tiles, and windowsills. Finally, a growing body of evidence suggests that cockroach allergens may be an important precipitant of asthma and rhinitis, especially in inner-city areas.[22,23]

Outdoor Allergens

Outdoor allergens vary widely with season and location but may be broadly divided into grasses, trees, and weeds.[21] Grass pollens are among the most frequent triggers of allergic symptoms, affecting 10% to 30% of allergic patients worldwide. Although many species of grass have been implicated in allergic disease, the allergenic proteins of most species have extensive immunologic cross-reactivity. As a result, mixtures of grass pollen extracts identify grass pollen-sensitive individuals, and there is seldom a need to test for each grass pollen individually because of this high degree of cross-reactivity. Exceptions include Johnson and Bermuda grasses, which are found primarily in the South and possess unique allergenic components.

Most tree pollens associated with allergy in North America are from deciduous trees, including birch, beech, oak, maple, elm, willow, poplar, aspen, olive, and ash trees. One coniferous tree, the mountain cedar, which is found in abundance in Texas and portions of the southwestern United States, also contributes substantially to seasonal allergic rhinitis and asthma. Tree pollen seasons typically occur in the early spring and usually are brief (4 to 6 weeks).

The main weed pollen in the United States is ragweed. There are two major forms of this plant, short ragweed (*Ambrosia artemisiaefolia*) and giant ragweed (*A trifida*), although other species are found in different locales throughout the United States. Other weeds that cause difficulty include *Amaranthus* and chenopods. The cross-reactivity of these weed pollens appears to be extensive, although some possess unique allergens.

A great number of fungi are allergenic, but the complexity of these allergens has hindered the development of standardized extracts.[21] Many of the extracts are of poor quality, and, with a few exceptions, justification for their use as either testing or treatment reagents is questionable. The most important species appear to be *Cladosporium*, *Alternaria*, *Aspergillus*, and *Penicillium*. *Alternaria* is primarily found outdoors and is a particularly potent allergen that has been linked to allergic rhinitis and asthma.[24]

Foods

Although food allergy can occur at any age, it is most common in young children who have respiratory, gastrointestinal, or dermatologic symptoms that appear soon after food ingestion.[25] The kinds of foods that cause allergic reactions vary with age: children are most often allergic to milk, eggs, soy, peanuts, or wheat, while adults are more likely to be allergic to seafood or nuts. In some instances, testing directly with fresh foods, such as a fruit or vegetable, by applying it to the skin and conducting a prick skin test may be useful.[26] Because of the high frequency of false-positive results with food skin tests, it is important to carefully correlate skin test results with data obtained from the history and food challenge test results before recommending dietary changes.[25]

Latex

Latex allergy is being recognized with increasing frequency, especially in high-risk groups such as health care workers, spina bifida patients, and other patients who have had increased latex exposure from repeated surgical procedures.[27] A well-defined latex skin test reagent has been tested in a multicenter study and appears to have good sensitivity and specificity.[28] Its approval by the Food and Drug Administration is pending. A RAST to detect latex-specific IgE is available, but false-negative tests are relatively common.

Risks of Skin Tests

Although skin testing is generally safe, anaphylactic reactions, including cases of fatal reactions, occur rarely.[29] To minimize the chance of severe adverse reactions, it is important to

Table 5: Controversial or Unproved Methods of Allergy Testing[35]

Procedures incapable of any measurement
- Cytotoxic tests
- Provocation/neutralization
- Electrodermal diagnosis
- Applied kinesiology
- Reaginic pulse test
- 'Body chemical' analysis

Valid tests that are inappropriate in the diagnosis of IgE-mediated allergy
- Allergen-specific IgG RAST or ELISA tests
- Immune complexes containing food proteins
- Certain measures of immunity
  - Quantitative IgG, IgA, IgM, IgD
  - Complement components
  - Lymphocyte subset analysis

Valid diagnostic allergy tests that are inappropriate for general use*
- Basophil histamine release
- In vitro lymphocyte proliferation

* These tests are often used in research protocols and may be indicated in certain clinical situations.

ensure the availability of a physician with the equipment and expertise to treat anaphylaxis and to evaluate patients for risk factors. Contraindications to skin testing include pregnancy, the presence of severe allergic symptoms, or the use of medications that block β-adrenergic receptors.[9]

Interpretation

Skin tests are interpreted by comparing the size of the wheal and flare responses to positive (histamine) or negative (diluent) controls. The tests may be scored using either qualitative (0 to 4+) or quantitative (diameter of wheal and flare in millimeters) measurements.[11] A prick test producing a wheal at least 3 mm larger than the negative control, or an intradermal test producing a wheal larger than 5 to 10 mm, usually indicates a clinically significant response. Results of RAST are usually expressed qualitatively in comparison to test results performed with a pool of serum from nonallergic individuals. Regardless of the scoring system, it is imperative that treatment recommendations not be based solely on results of skin tests or RAST.[30] Data pertaining to allergen-specific IgE must be correlated with a complete evaluation of allergen exposure, allergic symptoms, the physical examination, and the response to any previous medical therapy.

Unproved Methods of Allergy Testing

Many other tests are marketed as allergy tests or are used by 'alternative' health-care providers to diagnose allergy in patients who present with any of a variety of chronic health concerns (Table 5).[31-35] Some of these tests, such as measurement of T cell subsets by flow cytometry, are valid diagnostic tests but are of no value in the diagnosis of IgE-mediated allergic disorders. Other methods have never been rigorously tested or are of no value at all. Some tests are useful in allergy research or in a limited number of clinical scenarios, but their value as diagnostic procedures is limited by added costs or by a higher degree of precision than is warranted for general clinical use. To avoid results that may be misleading or of questionable significance, health-care providers should limit their diagnostic testing to methods of proven value in the clinical setting.[34,35]

Summary

Techniques such as skin testing or RAST, when used in conjunction with a careful evaluation of the history and physical examination, are an important part of the diagnostic evaluation of allergy. This information can dramatically improve treatment by allergen avoidance, medical management, and immunotherapy. The use of well-standardized testing procedures and careful quality control ensure that reliable data are provided, leading to sound clinical decisions.

References

1. Gergen PJ, Turkeltaub PC: The association of allergen skin test reactivity and respiratory disease among whites in the US population. Data from the Second National Health and Nutrition Examination Survey, 1976 to 1980. *Arch Intern Med* 1991;151:487-492.

2. Brand PL, Kerstjens HA, Jansen HM, et al: Interpretation of skin tests to house dust mite and relationship to other allergy parameters in patients with asthma and chronic obstructive pulmonary disease. The Dutch CNSLD Study Group. *J Allergy Clin Immunol* 1993;91:560-570.

3. Magnarin M, Knowles A, Ventura A, et al: A role for eosinophils in the pathogenesis of skin lesions in patients with food-sensitive atopic dermatitis. *J Allergy Clin Immunol* 1995;96:200-208.

4. Bousquet J, Chanez P, LaCoste JY, et al: Eosinophilic inflammation in asthma. *N Engl J Med* 1990;323:1033-1039.

5. Feather IH, Wilson SJ: Eosinophils in rhinitis. In: Busse WW, Holgate ST, eds. *Asthma and Rhinitis*. Cambridge, MA, Blackwell Scientific Publications, 1995, pp 347-363.

6. Jacobs RL, Freedman PM, Boswell RN: Nonallergic rhinitis with eosinophilia (NARES syndrome). Clinical and immunologic presentation. *J Allergy Clin Immunol* 1981;67:253-262.

7. Klink M, Cline MG, Halonen M, et al: Problems in defining normal limits for serum IgE. *J Allergy Clin Immunol* 1990; 85:440-444.

8. Sogn DD, Evans R 3d, Shepherd GM, et al: Results of the National Institute of Allergy and Infectious Diseases Collaborative Clinical Trial to test the predictive value of skin testing with major and minor penicillin derivatives in hospitalized adults. *Arch Intern Med* 1992;152:1025-1032.

9. Toogood JH: Risk of anaphylaxis in patients receiving beta-blocker drugs. *J Allergy Clin Immunol* 1988;81:1-5.

10. Erasmus C, Blackwood W, Wilson J: Infantile multicystic encephalomalacia after maternal bee sting anaphylaxis during pregnancy. *Arch Dis Child* 1982;57:785-787.

11. Yunginger JW, Ahlstedt S, Eggleston PA, et al: Quantitative IgE antibody assays in allergic diseases. *J Allergy Clin Immunol* 2000;105:1077-1084.

12. Ten RM, Klein JS, Frigas E: Allergy skin testing. *Mayo Clin Proc* 1995;70:783-784.

13. Nelson HS, Rosloniec DM, McCall LI, et al: Comparative performance of five commercial prick skin test devices. *J Allergy Clin Immunol* 1993;92:750-756.

14. Simons FE, Simons KJ: The pharmacology and use of H_1-receptor-antagonist drugs. *N Engl J Med* 1994;330:1663-1670.

15. Hamilton RG, Adkinson NF Jr: Clinical laboratory methods for the assessment and management of human allergic diseases. *Clin Lab Med* 1986;6:117-138.

16. Bush RK, Gern JE: Allergy evaluation: who, what and how. In: Schidlow DV, Smith DS, eds. *A Practical Guide to Pediatric Respiratory Diseases*. Philadelphia, Hanley & Belfus, 1994, pp 261-270.

17. Ownby DR, Adinoff AD: The appropriate use of skin testing and allergen immunotherapy in young children. *J Allergy Clin Immunol* 1994;94:662-665.

18. Duff AL, Platts-Mills TA: Allergens and asthma. *Pediatr Clin North Am* 1992;39:1277-1291.

19. Lindgren S, Belin L, Dreborg S, et al: Breed-specific dog-dandruff allergens. *J Allergy Clin Immunol* 1988;82:196-204.

20. Solomon WR, Platts-Mills TA: Aerobiology and inhalant allergens. In: Middleton E Jr, Reed CE, Ellis EF, et al, eds. *Allergy: Principles and Practice*. St. Louis, Mosby-Year Book, 1998, pp 367-403.

21. Bush RK: Fungal extracts in clinical practice. *Allergy Proc* 1993;14:385-390.

22. Garcia DP, Corbett ML, Sublett JL, et al: Cockroach allergy in Kentucky: a comparison of inner city, suburban, and rural small town populations. *Ann Allergy* 1994;72:203-208.

23. Kang BC, Johnson J, Veres-Thorner C: Atopic profile of inner-city asthma with a comparative analysis on the cockroach-

sensitive and ragweed-sensitive subgroups. *J Allergy Clin Immunol* 1993;92:802-811.

24. Perzanowski MS, Sporik R, Squillace SP, et al: Association of sensitization to *Alternaria* allergens with asthma among school-age children. *J Allergy Clin Immunol* 1998;101:626-632.

25. Sampson HA: Food allergy. *JAMA* 1997;278:1888-1894.

26. Rosen JP, Selcow JE, Mendelson LM, et al: Skin testing with natural foods in patients suspected of having food allergies: is it a necessity? *J Allergy Clin Immunol* 1994;93:1068-1070.

27. Slater JE: Latex allergy. *J Allergy Clin Immunol* 1994;94: 139-149.

28. Hamilton RG, et al: Diagnosis of natural rubber latex allergy: multicenter latex skin testing efficacy study. *J Allergy Clin Immunol* 1998;102:482-490.

29. Reid MJ, Lockey RF, Turkeltaub PC, et al: Survey of fatalities from skin testing and immunotherapy 1985-1989. *J Allergy Clin Immunol* 1993;92:6-15.

30. Nelson HS, Areson J, Reisman R: A prospective assessment of the remote practice of allergy: comparison of the diagnosis of allergic disease and the recommendations for allergen immunotherapy by board-certified allergists and a laboratory performing in vitro assays. *J Allergy Clin Immunol* 1993;92:380-386.

31. Condemi JJ: Unproved diagnostic and therapeutic techniques. In: Metcalfe DD, Sampson HA, Simon RA, eds. *Food Allergy: Adverse Reactions to Foods and Food Additives*. Boston, Blackwell Scientific Publications, 1997, pp 541-550.

32. VanArsdel PP Jr, Larson EB: Diagnostic tests for patients with suspected allergic disease. Utility and limitations. *Ann Intern Med* 1989;110:304-312.

33. Executive Committee of the American Academy of Allergy and Immunology: Clinical ecology. *J Allergy Clin Immunol* 1986;78:269-271.

34. American Academy of Allergy and Immunology: Unproven procedures for diagnosis and treatment of allergic and immunologic diseases. *J Allergy Clin Immunol* 1986;78:275-277.

35. Bernstein IL, Storms WW: Practice parameters for allergy diagnostic testing. *Ann Allergy Asthma Immunol* 1995;75(part II):553-625.

5

Allergic Conjunctivitis

Allergic eye symptoms are especially alarming to patients because, in addition to the annoying symptoms of itching and burning, the swelling and redness of the eyes are noticeable to family, friends, and coworkers. Consequently, when these symptoms occur, the health-care provider is expected to arrive at the correct diagnosis quickly and to prescribe fast-acting and effective remedies. This chapter reviews the diagnostic features of and treatments for the major forms of ocular allergy.

The three most common forms of ocular allergy are allergic rhinoconjunctivitis, atopic keratoconjunctivitis, and contact keratoconjunctivitis. Although these disorders are each associated with inflammation of the eyes and surrounding tissues, they can be distinguished by their clinical presentation (Table 1).

Allergic Rhinoconjunctivitis

Allergic rhinoconjunctivitis, also known as hay fever conjunctivitis, results from immunoglobulin E (IgE)-mediated inflammation of the conjunctiva triggered by outdoor allergens such as pollen or mold or by indoor allergens such as pet dander or house dust mite.[1] Symptoms include itching, redness, and tearing of the eyes, often accompanied

Table 1: Clinical Features of Allergic Eye Disease

	Allergic rhinoconjunctivitis
History	
Seasonal occurrence	Associated with pollen season and rhinitis symptoms
Atopic dermatitis	Sometimes
Pruritus	Yes
Discharge	Clear
Physical examination	
Pattern	Bilateral
Conjunctiva	Red and edematous, papillary response
Cornea	Usually not involved
Eyelid	Mild edema and redness with periocular edema
Cataracts	Unusual
Helpful adjuncts	
Skin tests or RAST	Yes
Patch tests	No
Conjunctival scrapings	Eosinophils

Atopic keratoconjunctivitis	Contact keratoconjunctivitis
Often worse in extremes of hot and cold weather	No
Yes	No
Yes	Yes
Stringy	+/-
Bilateral	Unilateral or bilateral, depending on mode of exposure
Red and edematous, Trantas' dots	Red, edematous (especially if caused by eyedrops)
May be involved	May be involved
Thickened with fissures, excoriations, scaling; especially upper lids	Erythema and edema prominent, papules or vesicles may be present
Develop after prolonged inflammation	Unusual
No	No
No	Yes
Eosinophils	Neutrophils, mononuclear cells, or eosinophils

by swelling about the eye. One of the cardinal features of allergic rhinoconjunctivitis is the coexistence of allergic rhinitis, and the severity of the nasal and ocular symptoms usually change in parallel. Pollen allergy is the most common trigger of allergic rhinoconjunctivitis, and symptoms usually occur at predictable times of the year, with peak symptoms usually limited to a few weeks. Many patients, however, are allergic to multiple pollens and thus experience the effects of several pollen seasons in series over the spring, summer, and fall. Patients allergic to indoor allergens usually have milder symptoms, but these may occur year-round, depending on the exposure. Patients allergic to animals can experience dramatic eye swelling and inflammation after contact with pets.

Physical findings include injection, erythema, and edema of the conjunctiva. The edema may sometimes be severe, producing chemosis, which is gross swelling of the bulbar conjunctiva. The palpebral conjunctiva may show a papillary response, consisting of erythema and fine polygonal papules from epithelial hypertrophy with inflammatory cell infiltration. The eyelids and the loose tissues below the eye may appear swollen, and the infraorbital region may have a bluish discoloration, producing 'allergic shiners.' The nasal mucosa is usually edematous, with increased mucoid secretions. The color of the mucosa varies: red, pale, or, with severe edema of the mucosa, bluish from venous congestion.

Most of the time, the history and physical examination provide sufficient information to make the diagnosis and initiate therapy, but allergy testing may be useful under several circumstances. First, skin testing or radioallergosorbent test (RAST) can help identify triggers for allergic symptoms so that efforts can be made to limit exposure to allergens in the home or work environment. Second, patients who have seasonal allergies and have not had a good response to medical therapy should be tested to confirm the diagnosis. The allergy test results can also be used to direct immunotherapy, if this is a consideration.

Treatment of allergic conjunctivitis is based on the same principles in treating allergic rhinitis (Chapter 6). If allergies are identified, efforts should be made to minimize allergen exposure, especially in the case of indoor allergens. Unfortunately, short of closing up the home or workspace and living in an air-conditioned environment, pollen is difficult to avoid, so medical therapy is necessary to control symptoms (Table 2).

Antihistamines, with or without decongestants, can provide quick relief of mild to moderate itching and redness of the eye. Although oral antihistamines (Table 2) provide adequate relief for many patients, topical antihistamines (eg, levocabastine [Livostin®]) provide more rapid relief (within minutes) and are generally more effective, although they require frequent administration.[2] Azelastine (Optivar®), ketotifen (Zaditor®), and olopatadine (Patanol®) are topical H_1-receptor blockers that also inhibit allergen-induced mast cell histamine release.[3,4] In addition to their effects on mast cells, ketotifen and azelastine inhibit eosinophil migration and mediator release.[5,6]

Topical nonsteroidal anti-inflammatory agents, such as ketorolac (Acular®), can be used to treat acute allergic symptoms, although they have few advantages over other classes of medications.[7] Patients with more severe rhinoconjunctivitis or who experience suboptimal relief with antihistamines alone may benefit from the use of a preventive medicine, such as lodoxamide (Alomide®) or nedocromil (Alocril®).[8,9] These mast cell stabilizing drugs are most effective when started before the onset of the pollen season and then continued daily for the duration of the season.[10]

In addition to medications, cool compresses can provide significant relief from pruritus and acute swelling. Nonmedicated artificial tears also provide symptomatic relief and can help to wash away the allergens and inflammatory mediators.

Additional measures are required for patients who experience unrelenting symptoms despite the measures discussed above. Corticosteroids are potent anti-inflammatory

Table 2: Medications for Allergic Eye Disease

Category	Medication
Topical Medications	
Artificial tears and lubricants	cellulose esters petrolatum polyvinyl alcohol
Vasoconstrictors	naphazoline HCl 0.01%-0.05% (Allerest®) tetrahydrozoline 0.05% (Visine®)
Antihistamines	levocabastine 0.05% (Livostin®) emedastine 0.05% (Emadine®)
Combination antihistamine/ vasoconstrictor	naphazoline 0.025%/ pheniramine 0.3% (Naphcon® A, Opcon® A)
Mast cell stabilizers	cromolyn 4% (Crolom®, Opticrom®) lodoxamide 0.1% (Alomide®) nedocromil 2% (Alocril®) pemirolast 0.1% (Almast®)
Antihistamine/ mast cell stabilizers	azelastine 0.05% (Optivar®) ketotifen 0.025% (Zaditor®) olopatadine 0.1% (Patanol®)
Nonsteroidal anti-inflammatories	ketorolac 0.5% (Acular®)
Glucocorticoids	loteprednol 0.2% (Alrex®, Lotemax®)

Dose	Comments
1 drop p.r.n. Small bead to lower eyelid p.r.n.	Blurred vision (especially ointments). Sensitivity to vehicle or preservatives may develop.
1 drop q.i.d. p.r.n.	Temporarily suppress redness, but rebound effect may occur after prolonged use.
1 drop q.i.d. p.r.n.	Rapid onset, but short duration.
1 drop q.i.d. p.r.n.	Approved for use in children ≥3 years.
1 drop q.i.d. p.r.n.	See above comments.
1 drop q.i.d. 1 drop q.i.d. 1 drop q.i.d. 1 drop q.i.d.	Best if started 1-2 weeks before and continued through the hay fever season. Approved for use in children ≥3 years.
1 drop b.i.d.	Approved for use in children ≥3 years.
1 drop q 8-12 h	Approved for use in children ≥3 years.
1 drop b.i.d. q 6-8 h	Approved for use in children ≥3 years.
1 drop q.i.d. p.r.n.	Use with caution in patients with bleeding disorders.
Begin with 1 drop q.i.d., taper to minimum effective dose	Prolonged use associated with glaucoma and cataracts; contraindicated in ocular herpes infection.

(continued)

Table 2: Medications for Allergic Eye Disease (continued)

Category	Medication
Oral Medications	
Antihistamines	
First-generation	diphenhydramine (Benadryl®)
	chlorpheniramine (Chlor-Trimeton®)
	hydroxyzine (Atarax®)
Second-generation	fexofenadine (Allegra®)
	cetirizine (Zyrtec®)
	desloratidine (Clarinex®)
	loratadine (Claritin®)
Corticosteroids	prednisone (Deltasone®)
	prednisolone (Pediapred®, Prelone®)

medications that are effective at relieving allergic inflammation when used topically or systemically. Although topical corticosteroids are safe when used in the nose, their chronic use in the eye can produce significant side effects, such as increased intraocular pressure or cataracts.[11] Also, the use of corticosteroids in an eye with herpetic infection can lead to extensive corneal ulceration and, ultimately, opacification. For these reasons, corticosteroid use in the eye should be minimized and, if necessary, used in collaboration with an ophthalmologist. Recently, 'soft' corticosteroids, such as loteprednol, have been shown to be effective in treating allergic conjunctivitis. Loteprednol (Alrex®, Lotemax®) may be less likely to cause side effects because

Dose	Comments
Short-acting or extended-release	Inexpensive, but side effects may limit clinical usefulness.
60 mg PO b.i.d. p.r.n.	Active metabolite of terfenadine.
5-10 mg PO q.d. p.r.n.	Incidence of sedation 11% 14%.
5 mg PO q.d. p.r.n.	
10 mg PO q.d. p.r.n.	
20 mg PO b.i.d. (adults) or 1 mg/kg/d (children) in split doses for 3-7 days	Very effective for quick relief of severe symptoms, but unsuitable for long-term use because of side effects.

it is rapidly metabolized in the anterior chamber. Even so, the lowest effective dose should be prescribed, and long-term use should be avoided.

Immunotherapy has proven to be an effective treatment for allergic rhinoconjunctivitis in carefully conducted clinical trials (Chapter 16).[12] In general, patients experience a one-third to one-half reduction in symptoms, which may make medical management easier or even unnecessary. Immunotherapy works better in patients with a few well-defined allergies, as opposed to those individuals who are 'allergic to everything.' Contraindications to immunotherapy include the use of a β-adrenergic blocking agent or the presence of severe or unstable asthma. Most patients derive

Table 3: Common Causes of Contact Allergy of the Eye

Eyedrops or ointments

- Antibiotics
  - neomycin
  - erythromycin
  - sulfacetamide
  - gentamicin
  - penicillin

- Other medications
  - benzocaine
  - pilocarpine
  - atropine
  - antazoline
  - phenylephrine
  - thimerosal
  - dorzolamide
  - apraclonidine

Other

- Occupational exposures
- Cosmetics
  - eyeliner
  - mascara
  - facial cream
- Fragrances
- Nail polish
- Hand creams
- Hairsprays

lasting benefits after 3 to 5 years of allergy injections, after which immunotherapy can usually be discontinued.[12]

Atopic Keratoconjunctivitis

Atopic dermatitis commonly involves the eyelids or cornea in adults and older children. This condition is known as atopic keratoconjunctivitis. Since allergic rhinoconjunctivitis and atopic keratoconjunctivitis are both found in atopic individuals, these conditions may coexist. The pathogenesis of atopic keratoconjunctivitis is thought to be similar to that of atopic dermatitis (Chapter 10) but has not been clearly defined. Biopsies of affected conjunctival tissue show increased numbers of mast cells, activated T lymphocytes, and goblet cells and stain positive for eosinophil granular proteins.[13] Although total and allergen-specific IgE levels are usually elevated in the serum and in tears,[14] allergies that are clearly related to the skin manifestations are the exception and not the rule.

Most patients with atopic keratoconjunctivitis have atopic dermatitis elsewhere on the body, although the ocular manifestations are sometimes the most prominent complaint.[15] Symptoms include pruritus, crusting in the morning, and redness. Corneal involvement may be heralded by photophobia. Physical findings include changes typical of atopic dermatitis, with thickened and red eyelids, accentuated skin lines, and small papular lesions that may be weepy or dry. Skin changes are usually most prominent on the upper eyelids. Scaling and lichenification appear with chronic lesions. The lid margins can appear thickened and scaly, with discharge that is most prominent in the early morning. The conjunctiva can be injected and edematous, with increased secretions, and scarring can develop after chronic inflammation. Trantas' dots, which are localized collections of eosinophils, may be present at the limbus. Corneal involvement, which can be detected by fluorescein staining, consists of punctate erosions. Patients with severe disease can also develop corneal scarring and keratoconus, a cone-shaped cornea thought to be associated with progressive corneal thinning.[16] Finally, cataracts can develop in atopic keratoconjunctivitis, most often in younger patients with severe and chronic disease.[17]

Eyelid dermatitis is treated the same as atopic dermatitis elsewhere on the face, with mild topical corticosteroid creams such as 1% hydrocortisone. The patient should be instructed to avoid getting the ointments into the eye itself. Blepharitis is treated with daily cleansing of the eyelids by gently scrubbing with baby shampoo or a mild soap to remove scales and crusting. Topical erythromycin ointment (Ilotycin®) will often eradicate local bacterial infection, which is heralded by an abrupt increase in erythema and discharge about the lid margins.

Conjunctival inflammation can be treated with regular application of cromolyn (Crolom®, Opticrom®) or lodoxamide. It is best to avoid long-term use of topical corticosteroids because of the high incidence of local complications.[11] Patients with corneal inflammation should be referred to an ophthalmologist for management. Contact lenses are available for the correction of keratoconus, but severe corneal involvement may require corneal transplantation.

Contact Keratoconjunctivitis

The skin of the eyelid and the surrounding area is thin and highly vascular and thus highly susceptible to contact dermatitis.[17] Sources of the allergen include eyedrops, cosmetics, and materials that first contact the hands and are then inoculated into the eyes by rubbing (Table 3). Because of the heightened sensitivity of the periocular tissues, the dermatopathology may be limited to the eyelids, even if the first contact with the allergen was via the hands. Contact keratoconjunctivitis is mediated by a type IV hypersensitivity reaction, and allergen-sensitized T lymphocytes are instrumental in producing the tissue inflammation.[18]

A common scenario for contact keratoconjunctivitis is a patient who is treated for an ocular condition with eyedrops, experiences transient improvement, and then develops intense itching, tearing, and redness of the eyes. Alternately, patients may experience similar symptoms without any clear trigger. On examination, the eyelids are usually very red and edematous, and microvesicles or shallow ulcers may be present. When eyedrops are involved, lower eyelid inflammation may be prominent, and the distribution of the dermatitis may correspond to the path of drops running down onto the face. The conjunctiva are usually intensely red, with a variable amount of edema. Severe cases may be accompanied by erosions of the corneal epithelium, which can be detected by fluorescein staining.

The diagnosis can often be made on the basis of typical physical findings that appear after the application of a known sensitizer, such as an ocular antibiotic or anesthetic. In cases of unclear origin, patch testing can help identify the allergen.[19] Treatment of contact allergy of the eye is to remove the inciting agent and to prevent future exposure to the allergen. Cool compresses can provide relief from mild or moderate swelling and itching, and short-term use of a mild topical corticosteroid agent (Table 2) or a short course of oral prednisone (Deltasone®) helps speed recovery in more severely affected individuals. Corticosteroid therapy is contraindicated if herpes infection of the eye is a consideration. For this reason, cases involving vesiculation of the eyelids, preauricular adenopathy, or corneal inflammation should be referred to an ophthalmologist for evaluation and treatment.

Vernal Keratoconjunctivitis

Vernal keratoconjunctivitis is a severe allergic eye disease that is limited to tropical climates and occurs mainly in young boys with allergic backgrounds.[20] As with hay fever conjunctivitis and atopic dermatitis, serum and local IgE levels are elevated, and conjunctival scrapings reveal increased numbers of activated T cells, eosinophils, and mast cells.[20-22] Allergy to house dust mite has been implicated in some cases.[17] The disorder typically appears in the preteen years and is active for 5 to 10 years before gradually resolving. The distinguishing feature of vernal keratoconjunctivitis is the development of severe allergic eye symptoms accompanied by a 'cobblestone' inflammation of the tarsal conjunctiva, consisting of many giant flat-topped papillae. These papillae can produce significant traumatic damage to the cornea, consisting of erosions or plaquelike deposits of epithelial cells in the anterior cornea.[23]

Treatment consists of providing symptomatic relief, as the disease is self-limited and has a good prognosis if corneal complications can be avoided.[17] Allergen avoidance may be helpful if dust mite or mold allergy is present. Medical therapy includes the use of mast cell stabilizing agents such as cromolyn or lodoxamide;[9] long-term use of corticosteroids should be avoided. Topical cyclosporine (Sandimmune®) has been helpful in some refractory cases.[24] The use of lubricating ointments (petrolatum) at night may help protect the cornea from traumatic damage.

Giant Papillary Conjunctivitis

Giant papillary conjunctivitis (GPC), a disorder found in wearers of soft contact lenses, has physical findings that resemble vernal conjunctivitis.[25] Although the mechanism underlying GPC is unknown, it is thought to be an immunologic reaction to the contact lens polymer or to a protein deposit on the lens material.[26] Gradual loss of meibomian glands is also observed in GPC, although it is not clear whether this is a cause or an effect of the disease.[27] Symptoms usually include redness, burning, itching, and discharge, which are relieved by removing the contacts for several days. Physical findings consist of redness of the conjunctiva, accompanied by a fine papillary response on the tarsal conjunctiva or large individual papillae in more chronic cases.

The most effective treatment for GPC is to discontinue wearing the contact lenses. For patients who desire to continue to wear contact lenses, disposable, daily-wear lenses are often well tolerated. The lens polymer is an important factor, because nonionic lenses with a low water content generally cause less inflammation.[25] Cromolyn eye drops may also be helpful for patients with GPC who wish to continue wearing contact lenses.[28]

Summary

Because of the presence of immunologically active tissue in the eye and the large degree of exposure to the environment, ocular allergy is one of the most frequently encountered complaints in a general office practice. Familiarity with the common forms of ocular allergy and their treatment enables the physician to provide effective therapy for these common diseases and to refer cases with potentially severe ocular complications to an ophthalmologist for further treatment.

References

1. Foster CS: The pathophysiology of ocular allergy: current thinking. *Allergy* 1995;50:6-9; (discussion) 34-38.

2. Sohoel P, Freng BA, Kramer J, et al: Topical levocabastine compared with orally administered terfenadine for the prophylaxis and treatment of seasonal rhinoconjunctivitis. *J Allergy Clin Immunol* 1993;92:73-81.

3. Olopatadine for allergic conjunctivitis. *Med Lett Drugs Ther* 1997;39:108-109.

4. Giede-Tuch C, Westhoff M, Zarth A: Azelastine eye-drops in seasonal allergic conjunctivitis. A double-blind, randomized, placebo-controlled study. *Allergy* 1998;53:857-862.

5. Ventura MT, Giuliano G, Di Corato R, et al: Modulation of eosinophilic chemotaxis with azelastine and budesonide in allergic patients. *Immunopharmacol Immunotoxicol* 1998;20:383-398.

6. Kato M, Hattori T, Takahashi M, et al: Eosinophil cationic protein and prophylactic treatment in pollinosis in natural allergen provocation. *Br J Clin Pract* 1994;48:299-301.

7. Ketorolac for seasonal allergic conjunctivitis. *Med Lett Drugs Ther* 1993;35:88-89.

8. Blumenthal M, Casale T, Dockhorn R, et al: Efficacy and safety of nedocromil sodium ophthalmic solution in the treatment of seasonal allergic conjunctivitis. *Am J Ophthalmol* 1992;113:56-63.

9. Lodoxamide for vernal keratoconjunctivitis. *Med Lett Drugs Ther* 1994;36:26.

10. Juniper EF, Guyatt GH, Ferrie PJ, et al: Sodium cromoglycate eye drops: regular versus "as needed" use in the treatment of seasonal allergic conjunctivitis. *J Allergy Clin Immunol* 1994;94: 36-43.

11. Friedlaender MH: Corticosteroid therapy of ocular allergy. *Int Ophthalmol Clin* 1983;23:175.

12. Durham SR, et al: Long-term clinical efficacy of grass pollen immunotherapy. *N Engl J Med* 1999;341:468-475.

13. Bielory L: Allergic and immunologic disorders of the eyes. Part II: ocular allergy. *J Allergy Clin Immunol* 2000;106:1019-1032.

14. Tuft SJ, Kemeny DM, Dart JK, et al: Clinical features of atopic keratoconjunctivitis. *Ophthalmology* 1991;98:150-158.

15. Akova YA, Jabbur NS, Neumann R, et al: Atypical ocular atopy. *Ophthalmology* 1993;100:1367-1371.

16. Donshik PC, Hoss DM, Ehlers WH: Inflammatory and papulosquamous disorders of the skin and eye. *Dermatol Clin* 1992; 10:533-547.

17. Bielory L: Allergic and immunologic disorders of the eye. In: Middleton E Jr, Reed CE, Ellis EF, et al, eds. *Allergy: Principles and Practice*. St. Louis, Mosby-Year Book, 1998, pp 1148-1161.

18. Kalish RS: Recent developments in the pathogenesis of allergic contact dermatitis. *Arch Dermatol* 1991;127:1558-1563.

19. Oshima H, Kawahara D, Hashimoto Y, et al: An approach to evaluating patch test results. *Contact Dermatitis* 1994;31:189-191.

20. Bonini S, Bonini S, Lambiase A, et al: Vernal keratoconjunctivitis: a model of 5q cytokine gene cluster disease. *Int Arch Allergy Immunol* 1995;107:95-98.

21. Maggi E, Biswas P, Del Prete G, et al: Accumulation of Th-2-like helper T cells in the conjunctiva of patients with vernal conjunctivitis. *J Immunol* 1991;146:1169-1174.

22. Trocme SD, Kephart GM, Bourne WM, et al: Eosinophil granule major basic protein deposition in corneal ulcers associated with vernal keratoconjunctivitis. *Am J Ophthalmol* 1993; 115:640-643.

23. Cameron JA: Shield ulcers and plaques of the cornea in vernal keratoconjunctivitis. *Ophthalmology* 1995;102:985-993.

24. Kaan G, Ozden O: Therapeutic use of topical cyclosporine. *Ann Ophthalmol* 1993;25:182-186.

25. Donshik PC: Giant papillary conjunctivitis. *Trans Am Ophthalmol Soc* 1994;92:687-744.

26. Meisler DM, Keller WB: Contact lens type, material, and deposits and giant papillary conjunctivitis. *CLAO J* 1995;21:77-80.

27. Mathers WD, Billborough M: Meibomian gland function and giant papillary conjunctivitis. *Am J Ophthalmol* 1992;114: 188-192.

28. Kruger CJ, Ehlers WH, Luistro AE, et al: Treatment of giant papillary conjunctivitis with cromolyn sodium. *CLAO J* 1992; 18:46-48.

6

Allergic Rhinitis

llergic rhinitis is the most common form of respiratory allergy, affecting 15% to 20% of the general population, and, like asthma, its prevalence is increasing for reasons that are unclear.[1,2] Allergic rhinitis is primarily an affliction of children and young adults. Symptoms can appear as early as infancy; prevalence is greatest during the teenage years and the early 20s and decreases thereafter.[1] Although many individuals with allergic rhinitis have limited symptoms, allergic rhinitis can be incapacitating during the peak pollen seasons. Despite the availability of safe and effective remedies, a large segment of the population is undertreated and continues to suffer through the allergy seasons with only marginally effective over-the-counter remedies.[3]

Diagnosis

The signs and symptoms of allergic rhinitis are well known to most health-care providers (Table 1), and making the diagnosis of seasonal allergic rhinitis or hay fever is usually straightforward. Symptoms such as nasal congestion, rhinorrhea, nasal itching, and sneezing that occur seasonally strongly support the diagnosis of allergic rhinitis. Associated problems may include allergic conjunctivitis,

Table 1: Clinical Presentation of Allergic Rhinitis

Symptoms	Signs	Complications
• Nasal congestion	• Swollen nasal mucosa: pale, bluish, or red	• Allergic conjunctivitis
• Rhinorrhea	• Rhinorrhea	• Otitis media
• Nasal itching	• Lymphoid aggregates on mucous membranes	• Sinusitis
• Loss of taste and smell		• Sleep disturbances
• Itching of the soft palate	• Dennie's lines	
• Sneezing	• Allergic salute	
• Headache	• Nasal crease	
	• Serous middle ear effusion	

otitis media, sinusitis, loss of taste or smell, sleep disturbances, and headache. Physical findings can include puffy, red eyes, swollen nasal mucosa that may be pale, bluish, or even red, nasal discharge that is usually clear and thin, serous effusion in the middle ears, and lymphoid aggregates on the soft palate and posterior pharynx. Other telltale signs of allergic rhinitis include extra skin folds under the lower eyelids (Dennie's lines) and a crease on the anterior third of the nose from frequent nasal itching.

These stereotypical signs and symptoms of allergic rhinitis are usually sufficient to arrive at the correct diagnosis. However, laboratory testing to confirm the clinical suspicion may be useful when symptoms are perennial instead of seasonal or when patients do not respond favorably to standard treatment regimens. Allergy testing also

Table 2: Testing for Allergic Rhinitis

- Allergen-specific IgE
  - RAST
  - Skin tests (prick or intradermal)
- Total serum IgE–poor sensitivity and specificity
- Nasal smear for eosinophils

provides important preventive information that can be used to guide recommendations about allergen avoidance (see Chapter 16). This is especially important in the case of sensitization to indoor allergens such as animals, house dust mites, and mold.[4,5]

Testing for respiratory allergy is based on the detection of allergen-specific immunoglobulin E (IgE) (Table 2). Both radioallergosorbent test (RAST) and skin tests provide data that are comparable in terms of sensitivity and specificity. The choice of which test to use depends largely on availability, but a few other factors need to be considered.[6] Skin tests yield information within a few minutes and are relatively inexpensive, but the results are strongly influenced by the quality of the allergenic extracts employed, the technique used to perform the skin tests, and the condition of the skin. In addition, antihistamine use must be discontinued for skin testing to be performed. RAST is also influenced by technical factors and must be sent to a reputable laboratory. These tests are relatively expensive but are widely available, and results are not influenced by the presence of antihistamines. In contrast to the clinical utility of measuring allergen-specific IgE, total serum IgE is not useful in evaluating patients with suspected allergic rhinitis because of the large degree of overlap between total serum IgE levels in allergic and nonallergic individuals.[6,7]

Finally, examining nasal secretions for eosinophilia can help in evaluating patients with chronic rhinitis. A nasal smear is prepared by having the patient blow his or her nose into a sheet of plastic wrap, transferring the secretions to a microscope slide, allowing it to air dry, and then staining the slide with either Hansel's or Giemsa stain. The presence of greater than 25% eosinophils suggests respiratory allergy, although this may also indicate nonallergic rhinitis with eosinophilia (NARES).[8]

Treatment

Three modes of therapy are effective for treating allergic rhinitis: allergen avoidance, medical therapy, and immunotherapy/allergen desensitization (Figure 1).

Allergen avoidance is an effective means of preventing symptoms triggered by indoor allergies such as house dust mite, animals, or mold (see Chapter 16).[9] However, it is difficult to avoid airborne pollens without reverting to a reclusive, air-conditioned lifestyle during warm-weather months. Symptoms that persist despite allergen avoidance are treated with medical therapy, which is directed at the underlying inflammation of the nasal mucosa and at inhibition of mediators such as histamine.[10,11] The combination of a topical corticosteroid nasal spray and an oral antihistamine produces a good clinical response in most patients, although patients with mild symptoms may do well with an antihistamine alone.

Antihistamines were considered a first-line treatment against allergic rhinitis for many years, and newer agents have a longer duration of action and few side effects. However, it is now clear that histamine is only one of many mediators causing allergic rhinitis symptoms,[12] and thus antihistamines provide only partial symptom relief for most patients. In general, antihistamines are effective for treatment of sneezing, itching, and rhinorrhea, but have relatively little effect on congestion, which is one of the most troublesome symptoms of allergic rhinitis.[13] First-genera-

84

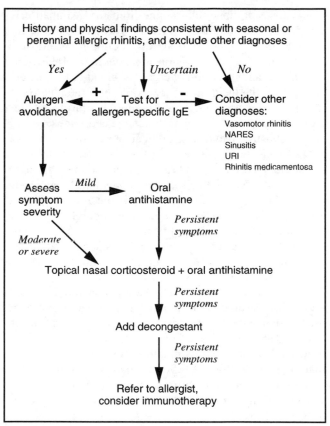

Figure 1: Overview of the diagnosis and treatment of allergic rhinitis.

tion antihistamines are effective histamine blockers but produce clinically apparent sedation in about one third of users. Recent studies using neuropsychologic testing or electroencephalographic monitoring have demonstrated that first-generation antihistamines produce subtle central nervous system effects in most patients.[14,15] In addition, tests conducted in a driving simulator indicate that therapeutic doses of diphenhydramine (Benadryl®) impair driving performance and that effects were comparable to a blood alcohol level of 0.01% (legal definition of intoxication).[16] The second-generation antihistamines (Table 3) are lipophobic, and most do not cross the blood-brain barrier.[13] As a result, the incidence of sedation for loratadine (Claritin®), fexofenadine (Allegra®), and desloratidine (Clarinex®) is no greater than placebo, while cetirizine (Zyrtec®) and acrivastine (Semprex-D®) cause sedation in 10% to 15% of patients. These newer antihistamines also have relatively long half-lives and retain potent antihistaminic effects. Finally, azelastine (Astelin®), a potent H_1-antihistamine and mast cell stabilizer, is available as a nasal spray. This topical antihistamine provides prompt relief of sneezing and nasal itching, has a low incidence (11.5%) of sedation, and can be used in children 3 years of age and older.[17] These medications can be used either intermittently for symptom relief or prophylactically.[15]

Although they are generally safe, some antihistamines may cause cardiac arrhythmias when taken in overdose, used in standard doses by patients with liver disease or prolonged QTc interval, or taken in conjunction with medications such as erythromycin and ketoconazole (Nizoral®) that interfere with the P-450 microsomal system.[13] Fexofenadine, loratadine, cetirizine, and acrivastine do not produce cardiac side effects because they do not prolong the QTc interval.[13]

One common misconception is that antihistamines should not be used in patients with asthma, and this error has been reinforced by long-standing, but mistaken, warnings on package inserts. In fact, good control of allergic rhinitis with antihistamines and topical nasal corticosteroids can actually improve control of lower airway symptoms in patients with asthma.[4] Antihistamines are often combined in drug mixtures with decongestants that may counteract the sedative effect of antihistamines to some degree and potentiate the decongestive effects of the antihistamine.[18] Oral decongestants are α-adrenergic agonists that act by constricting blood vessels in the nasal mucosa but can also cause side effects, such as tremor, insomnia, and nervousness.[19] Oral decongestants can also aggravate certain other medical conditions, such as restricting urinary flow in males, and they are contraindicated in patients with hypertension or glaucoma.[19,20]

Topical corticosteroid nasal sprays are the single most effective treatment for allergic rhinitis symptoms (Table 4). These medications relieve a wide range of symptoms and have a low incidence of side effects. Local side effects, such as mucosal atrophy and nosebleeds, occur in less than 5% of patients. In children treated with beclomethasone nasal spray or metered-dose inhaler, small but measurable effects on growth have been noted. Beclomethasone topical therapy appears to reduce the rate of growth by 1 to 1.5 cm in the first year.[21,22] Because studies suggest that the eventual attained height of children treated with topical corticosteroids is normal, it is assumed that the effect on growth is temporary and that catch-up growth does occur.[23] Even so, low-dose topical therapy with mometasone (Nasonex®) or fluticasone (Flonase®), which are more rapidly metabolized, has not been associated with growth delay,[24,25] and these may be the preferred medications for treating allergic rhinitis in children.

Because few studies compare the different corticosteroid medications head to head, the choice of which spray to prescribe for a particular patient is largely one of personal preference. Differentiating features include dry vs wet sprays and scented vs unscented formulations. Several of the topical corticosteroids are particularly easy to use because they can be administered once daily. Regardless of which preparation is selected, corticosteroid sprays are most effective when used prophylactically, and using them intermittently may produce suboptimal clinical responses.[26] To derive maximum benefit, it is best to start topical nasal corticosteroid therapy 1 or 2 weeks before the start of an al-

Table 3: Second-Generation Antihistamines

Medication	Brand name	Recommended dose
acrivastine	Semprex-D®	8 mg PO q 4-6 h
cetirizine	Zyrtec®	5-10 mg PO q.d. (ages 6 years and older)
	Zyrtec-D 12-Hour™	5 mg PO b.i.d.
desloratidine	Clarinex®	5 mg PO q.d.
fexofenadine	Allegra®	30 mg PO b.i.d. (ages 6 to 11 years) 60 mg PO b.i.d. (ages 12 years and older) 180 mg PO q.d. (ages 12 years and older)
	Allegra-D™	60 mg PO b.i.d.
loratadine	Claritin®	5 mg PO q.d. (ages 2 to 6 years) 10 mg PO q.d. (ages 6 years and older)
	Claritin®–D 12 Hour	5 mg PO b.i.d.
	Claritin®–D 24 Hour	10 mg PO q.d.

How supplied

Comments

Capsules containing
8 mg acrivastine and
60 mg pseudoephedrine

- Incidence of sedation 12%
- Relatively short half-life
- Does not increase QTc
- Capsules also contain 60 mg
  pseudoephedrine

5-mg, 10-mg tablets
5-mg/tsp syrup
5 mg cetirizine and
120 mg pseudoephedrine

- Metabolite of hydroxyzine
- Incidence of sedation 11% to 14%
- Does not increase QTc

5-mg tablets

- Does not increase QTc
- Incidence of sedation similar
  to placebo

60 mg capsules
30, 60, and
180 mg tablets

- Metabolite of terfenadine
- Incidence of sedation
  similar to placebo
- Does not increase QTc

60 mg fexofenadine and
120 mg pseudoephedrine

10-mg tablets
5 mg/tsp syrup

10 mg rapidly
disintegrating tablets

- Does not increase QTc
- Incidence of sedation
  similar to placebo
- Freeze-dried tablet that
  dissolves on the tongue
  and can be taken without water

5 mg loratadine and
120 mg pseudoephedrine

10 mg loratadine and
240 mg pseudoephedrine

- Only once-daily combination agent
- Low incidence of insomnia (5%)

Table 4: Topical Nasal Corticosteroid Preparations

Medication	Brand name	μg/puff
beclomethasone	Beconase AQ®	42
	Vancenase Pockethaler®	42
	Vancenase AQ®	84
budesonide	Rhinocort Aqua®	32
flunisolide	Nasarel®	25
fluticasone	Flonase®	50
mometasone	Nasonex®	50
triamcinolone	Nasacort®	55
	Nasacort AQ®	

*If a positive clinical response occurs, titrate the dose downward to determine the lowest daily dose that provides adequate relief of symptoms.

Recommended dose*

Pediatric**		Adult		
Spray(s) per nostril	µg/d	Spray(s) per nostril	µg/d	Comments
1 b.i.d. (1-2 b.i.d.)	168-336	**1 b.i.d.** (1-2 b.i.d.)	168-336	Aqueous spray
1 t.i.d.	252	**1 b.i.d.-q.i.d.**	168-336	Dry spray
1 q.d. (1-2 q.d.)	168-336	**1 q.d.** (1-2 q.d.)	168-336	Aqueous spray
1 q.d. (1-2 q.d.)	64-128	**1 q.d.** (1-4 q.d.)	64-256	Unscented aqueous spray
2 b.i.d. or 1 t.i.d.	150-200	**2 b.i.d.**	200-400	Aqueous spray
		(2 b.i.d.-q.i.d.)	200-400	
1 q.d. (1-2 q.d.)	100-200	**2 q.d.** (1-2 q.d.)	100-200	Aqueous spray approved for patients ≥4 years of age
1 q.d.	100	**2 q.d.**	200	Aqueous spray approved for patients ≥2 years of age
2 q.d.	220	**2 q.d.-b.i.d.**	200-440	Dry spray
1 q.d. (1-2 q.d.)	110-220	**2 q.d.**	220	Unscented aqueous spray

**6 years of age and older unless otherwise noted

Boldface: Recommended starting dose

Dosage range shown in parentheses.

Table 5: Technique for Administering Topical Nasal Spray

- Shake canister and remove the cover.
  Pump sprays must be 'primed' before the first use of a new bottle by pumping the sprayer 2-4 times until a uniform spray is produced.

- Blow your nose to clear the airway.

- Insert the nosepiece of the inhaler just inside one nostril. Aim the tip away from the nasal septum and toward the ipsilateral earlobe.

- Activate inhaler while gently inspiring through the nose.

- Spray the other nostril, and repeat as directed.

lergy season. Although these medications have an excellent safety record, patients who use nasal corticosteroid preparations daily should have a nasal examination performed every 6 to 12 months because atrophy or ulceration of the nasal mucosa can occur with overuse or improper administration technique.

Topical cromolyn sodium (Nasalcrom®) also has anti-inflammatory properties and an excellent safety record and is now available without a prescription. However, topical cromolyn is less effective than nasal corticosteroids,[27] has the disadvantage of high cost, and requires frequent administration (3 to 4 times a day).

When prescribing nasal inhalers, the prescribing physician or one of the clinic staff must review with the patient the instructions for proper medication administration (Table 5). Moreover, the patient must demonstrate proper technique during the clinic visit. Do not assume that patients will learn the proper method for administration by reading the package insert! Improper use of topical corticosteroids can increase the frequency of side effects such as nose-bleeds and reduce the efficacy of these medications.

Patients who suffer severe nasal symptoms during the pollen allergy season, especially those who present with completely occluded nasal passageways, may benefit significantly by taking a short course of an oral corticosteroid (eg, prednisone 20 mg PO b.i.d. x 5 days in adolescents or adults). This accomplishes two goals: prompt and dramatic clinical relief and opening of the airway so that topical nasal sprays can reach the target tissues. Although short courses of oral corticosteroids rarely cause serious side effects, corticosteroid therapy may cause problems in patients with complicating health problems such as hypertension or diabetes.

Topical vasoconstrictors such as oxymetazoline (Afrin®) and phenylephrine (Neo-Synephrine®) have been heavily marketed for the treatment of upper respiratory infections and allergic symptoms. Because of the possibility of rebound congestion that occurs after only a few days of continuous use in some patients, topical vasoconstrictors are not suitable for use in allergic rhinitis patients, whose symptoms may last several weeks or months.

Two other classes of medications may also be useful in treating chronic rhinitis. The leukotriene receptor antagonists and synthesis inhibitors constitute a new class of oral antiallergic medications. These medicines were primarily developed to treat asthma but also relieve allergic nasal symptoms.[28] The place of these medications in the treatment of allergic rhinitis remains to be defined. Anticholinergic nasal sprays such as ipratropium bromide (Atrovent®) act directly on the secretory glands of the nose to decrease the production of nasal secretions. These medications represent a major advance in the treatment of vasomotor rhinitis[29] but will probably contribute little to the control of allergic rhinitis managed with topical corticosteroids and oral antihistamines.

Finally, immunotherapy is another allergic rhinitis treatment with proven efficacy. Although allergy specialists have different opinions about when to recommend immunotherapy, it is probably best used in patients who do not respond favorably to the combination of allergen avoidance and medications. Double-blind, placebo-controlled trials have shown that immunotherapy can produce long-lasting relief of allergic rhinitis symptoms triggered by pollens, house dust mites, molds,[30,31] and, in some cases, pets.

Summary

Because allergic rhinitis is one of the most common symptoms prompting outpatient clinic visits, health-care providers of every specialty need to be familiar with the presenting signs, symptoms, and therapy for this bothersome disorder. Topical corticosteroid preparations and the newer antihistamines provide effective relief of rhinitis symptoms, with low instances of side effects and a good safety record. Patients who do not respond to the combination of allergen avoidance and medical therapy should be referred to an allergist for further evaluation and to consider the possibility of treatment with immunotherapy.

References

1. Sibbald B, Strachan DP: Epidemiology of rhinitis. In: Busse WW, Holgate ST, eds. *Asthma and Rhinitis*. Cambridge, MA, Blackwell Scientific Publications, 1995, pp 32-43.

2. Fleming DM, Crombie DL: Prevalence of asthma and hay fever in England and Wales. *Br Med J (Clin Res Ed)* 1987;294:279-283.

3. Richards S, Thornhill D, Roberts H, et al: How many people think they have hay fever, and what they do about it. *Br J Gen Pract* 1992;42:284-286.

4. Bousquet J, Van Cauwenberge P, Khaltaev N, et al: Allergic rhinitis and its impact on asthma: ARIA Workshop Report. *J Allergy Clin Immunol* 2001;108(5 Suppl):S147-S334.

5. Fernandez-Caldas E, Trudeau WL, Ledford DK: Environmental control of indoor biologic agents. *J Allergy Clin Immunol* 1994; 94:404-412.

6. Bush RK, Gern JE: Allergy evaluation: who, what and how. In: Schidlow DV, Smith DS, eds. *A Practical Guide to Pediatric Respiratory Diseases*. Philadelphia, Hanley & Belfus, 1994, pp 261-270.

7. Klink M, Cline MG, Halonen M, et al: Problems in defining normal limits for serum IgE. *J Allergy Clin Immunol* 1990; 85:440-444.

8. Mullarkey MF, Hill JS, Webb DR: Allergic and nonallergic rhinitis: their characterization with attention to the meaning of nasal eosinophilia. *J Allergy Clin Immunol* 1980;65:122-126.

9. Platts-Mills TA, Vaughan JW, Carter MC, et al: The role of intervention in established allergy: avoidance of indoor allergens in the treatment of chronic allergic disease. *J Allergy Clin Immunol* 2000;106:787-804.

10. Naclerio RM: Allergic rhinitis. *N Engl J Med* 1991;325: 860-869.

11. Pipkorn U, Pukander J, Suonpaa J, et al: Long-term safety of budesonide nasal aerosol: a 5.5-year follow-up study. *Clin Allergy* 1988;18:253-259.

12. Naclerio RM, Proud D, Togias AG, et al: Inflammatory mediators in late antigen-induced rhinitis. *N Engl J Med* 1985; 313:65-70.

13. Simons FE, Simons KJ: The pharmacology and use of H_1-receptor-antagonist drugs. *N Engl J Med* 1994;330:1663-1670.

14. Bender B, Milgrom H: Neuropsychiatric effects of medications for allergic diseases. *J Allergy Clin Immunol* 1995; 95:523-528.

15. Simons FE: The eternal triangle: benefit, risk, and cost of therapeutic agents. *Ann Allergy Asthma Immunol* 1996;77:337-340.

16. Weiler JM, Bloomfield JR, Woodworth GG, et al: Effects of fexofenadine, diphenhydramine, and alcohol on driving performance. A randomized, placebo-controlled trial in the Iowa driving simulator. *Ann Intern Med* 2000;132:354-363.

17. Azelastine nasal spray for allergic rhinitis. *Med Lett Drugs Ther* 1997;39:45-47.

18. Falliers CJ, Redding MA: Controlled comparison of a new antihistamine-decongestant combination to its individual components. *Ann Allergy* 1980;45:75-80.

19. Druce HM: Allergic and nonallergic rhinitis. In: Middleton E Jr, Reed CE, Ellis EF, et al, eds. *Allergy: Principles and Practice*. St. Louis, Mosby-Year Book, 1998, pp 1005-1016.

20. Chua SS, Benrimoj SI, Gordon RD, et al: A controlled clinical trial on the cardiovascular effects of single doses of pseudoephedrine in hypertensive patients. *Br J Clin Pharmacol* 1989; 28:369-372.

21. Skoner DP, Rachelefsky GS, Meltzer ED, et al: Detection of growth suppression in children during treatment with intranasal beclomethasone dipropionate. *Pediatrics* 2000;105:E23.

22. Simons FE: A comparison of beclomethasone, salmeterol, and placebo in children with asthma. Canadian Beclomethasone Dipropionate-Salmeterol Xinafoate Study Group. *N Engl J Med* 1997;337:1659-1665.

23. Agertoft L, Pedersen S: Effect of long-term treatment with inhaled budesonide on adult height in children with asthma. *N Engl J Med* 2000;343:1064-1069.

24. Allen DB, Bronsky EA, Laforce CF, et al: Growth in children treated with fluticasone propionate. *J Pediatr* 1998;132:472-477.

25. Schenkel EJ, Skoner DP, Bronsky EA, et al: Absence of growth retardation in children with perennial allergic rhinitis after one year of treatment with mometasone furoate aqueous nasal spray. *Pediatrics* 2000;105:E22.

26. Juniper EF, Guyatt GH, Archer B, et al: Aqueous beclomethasone dipropionate in the treatment of ragweed pollen-induced rhinitis: further exploration of "as needed" use. *J Allergy Clin Immunol* 1993;92:66-72.

27. Welsh PW, Stricker WE, Chu CP, et al: Efficacy of beclomethasone nasal solution, flunisolide, and cromolyn in relieving symptoms of ragweed allergy. *Mayo Clin Proc* 1987;62:125-134.

28. Knapp HR: Reduced allergen-induced nasal congestion and leukotriene synthesis with an orally active 5-lipoxygenase inhibitor. *N Engl J Med* 1990;323:1745-1748.

29. Grossman J, Banov C, Boggs P, et al: Use of ipratropium bromide nasal spray in chronic treatment of nonallergic perennial rhinitis, alone and in combination with other perennial rhinitis medications. *J Allergy Clin Immunol* 1995;95:1123-1127.

30. Weber RW: Immunotherapy with allergens. *JAMA* 1997; 278:1881-1887.

31. Durham SR, et al: Long-term efficacy of grass pollen immunotherapy. *N Engl J Med* 1999;341:468-475.

7

Asthma

lthough asthma has always been a common medical problem, its prevalence and severity have increased worldwide over the past 20 years. This trend
has coincided with an explosion of knowledge about the
pathogenesis of asthma, which has led to the development of
new and more effective treatment strategies. In this chapter,
we will outline the diagnostic evaluation of asthma and the
development of treatment regimens that are individualized
according to specific triggers of acute symptoms and to the
severity of disease. Much of the information in this chapter
is based on reports from two expert panels that recently con-
vened to distill advances in asthma research into practical
guidelines for asthma diagnosis and management.[1,2]

Definition

Asthma was long defined as reversible obstructive airway disease caused by abnormal control of the airway
smooth muscle. Recent studies of asthma pathophysiology,
especially those using direct sampling of lower airway cells
or secretions by flexible bronchoscopy, have expanded the
definition of asthma to include the concepts of chronic inflammation and airway hyperresponsiveness (Figure 1,
Table 1).[1,2] Both these features of asthma have been linked

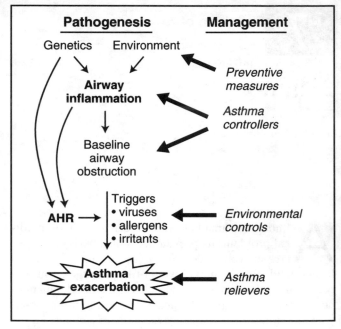

Figure 1: Overview of the pathogenesis of asthma.
AHR = airway hyperresponsiveness.

to specific genes, including cytokine genes that regulate
mucosal immune response to allergens, and to environmental factors such as exposure to allergens, tobacco smoke,
and the Western industrialized lifestyle.[1-3] The principal
pathologic finding in asthma is the infiltration of the lower
respiratory mucosa and secretions with inflammatory cells
such as eosinophils, mast cells, and activated T lymphocytes.[4] The mediators and cytokines secreted by these cells
cause many of the hallmark features of asthma, including
damage to airway epithelial cells, edema of the airway mucosa, hypersecretion of mucus, neural irritation, and airway
hyperresponsiveness. Airway hyperresponsiveness, which
is found in nearly all patients with asthma, is defined as an

Table 1: Definition of Asthma

- Variable airway obstruction
- Airway inflammation
- Airway hyperresponsiveness

increased susceptibility to bronchoconstriction that may be triggered by physical stimuli (exercise, cold air), irritants (tobacco smoke), or allergens.[5] In addition, viral upper respiratory infections are frequent triggers of acute exacerbations of asthma in adults and children.[6] Finally, chronic airway inflammation can lead to thickening of the basement membrane and deposition of collagen in the bronchial wall. This remodeling of airway structures contributes to chronic small-airway obstruction in asthma and may eventually lead to irreversible chronic obstructive pulmonary disease.[7]

Diagnosing Asthma

The diagnosis of asthma is based on the patient's medical history and physical examination, and objective measurements of pulmonary function (Figure 2). The medical history should include a description of the character and pattern of respiratory symptoms, triggers for symptoms, and any medications (over-the-counter or prescribed) used to treat symptoms (Table 2). Cough, wheezing, or dyspnea that worsen in the early morning hours or with exercise are typical complaints. In addition to inquiring about exercise-induced symptoms, clinicians must also determine whether asthma limits a patient's exercise or affects school or job performance. For example, someone who consistently wheezes with exercise may consciously or unconsciously decide to stop exercising.

Family and social histories are relevant to the diagnosis and treatment of asthma. There is no question that heredity plays a role in asthma pathogenesis. Most asthmatic patients

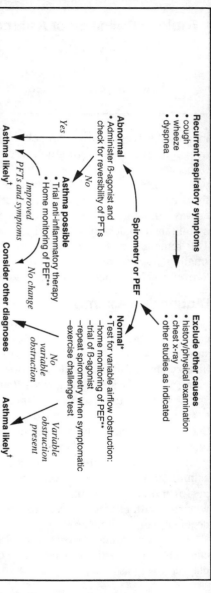

Figure 2: Diagnostic evaluation of asthma.
*Peak expiratory flow (PEF) in the 'normal' range may in fact be low for an individual whose lung function is usually above average. In this regard, spirometry can provide additional information (eg, FEV₁/FVC ratio) helpful in recognizing airway obstruction. If PEF is 'normal' and spirometry is not available, consider testing for improvement of PEF after administration of a β-adrenergic agonist.
**Monitor PEF during asymptomatic and symptomatic periods for 1 to 2 weeks. If the PEF is low, document the response of PEF and symptoms to inhaled β-adrenergic agonist.
†Institute therapy and reevaluate in 1 month.

Table 2: Asthma: Important Aspects of the Medical History

Symptoms
- Coughing, wheezing, shortness of breath, modest sputum production
- Often worse at night
- Response to bronchodilators

Triggers
- Upper respiratory infection
- Allergen exposure (pets, house dust, pollens)
- Work-related exposures
- Irritants (tobacco smoke)
- Exercise
- Cold air
- Emotions

Disease course
- Age of onset and diagnosis
- Response to previous treatments
- Hospitalizations, intensive care unit or emergency room visits

Impact of disease on patient or family
- School or workdays missed
- Limitation of exercise
- Nocturnal awakenings
- Psychologic effects

have relatives with asthma, respiratory allergies, or eczema.[8] Previous family experiences with asthma may strongly influence a patient's own attitude toward treatment. Exposure to environmental factors associated with asthma, such as pets,

Table 3: Risk Factors for Asthma Mortality

Age
- Elderly
- Teenagers

Ethnicity
- African Americans

Hospital admissions
- Intubation
- Intensive care unit admission

Underestimation of asthma severity
- Poor recognition of asthma symptoms
- Inadequate treatment
- Overuse of inhaled bronchodilators

Psychologic factors
- Depression

Low socioeconomic status
- Lack of access to medical care

Alternaria *allergy*

molds, tobacco smoke, and occupational irritants or allergens, should also be elicited. Risk factors for particularly severe exacerbations should be identified. These risk factors may reflect severe asthma, socioeconomic hindrances, or a combination of these factors (Table 3) and will identify patients with special treatment needs.[9,10]

If the medical history suggests the possibility of asthma, particular attention should be paid to the examination of the chest, upper respiratory tract, and skin. Wheezing of the chest is one of the main characteristics of asthma, but because airway obstruction in asthma is often erratic, examination of the chest during regular visits is often normal. It is important to note that wheezing may be absent even with moderate (up to 25% reduction in peak expiratory flow [PEF]) airway obstruction[11] and during severe exacerbations of asthma when airflow is severely limited. Other physical findings associated with asthma are the use of accessory muscles during tidal breathing, a prolonged expiratory phase, and a barrel-chested appearance. Physical examination may also reveal signs of coexistent atopic diseases, such as allergic rhinitis, allergic conjunctivitis, or atopic dermatitis. The presence of nasal polyps suggests aspirin hypersensitivity[12] or cystic fibrosis.[13] Clubbing of the fingers is not characteristic of asthma and suggests either heart disease or other chronic respiratory conditions such as bronchiectasis or cystic fibrosis.

Patients whose history and physical findings suggest asthma should be further evaluated with objective measurements of pulmonary function. A spirometer is a wise investment for any health-care practitioner who regularly cares for patients with asthma. Measurements that suggest obstruction of the small airways include reduction in forced expiratory volume in 1 second (FEV_1), in PEF, in the ratio of FEV_1 to forced vital capacity (FEV_1/FVC ratio), or in the midexpiratory forced expiratory flow rate (FEF_{25-75}).[1,2] For patients with evidence of airway obstruction, a β-adrenergic agonist should be administered either via metered-dose inhaler (MDI) or nebulizer, and pulmonary function tests (PFTs) should be repeated 15 to 30 minutes later to determine whether the abnormalities are reversible. An increase in PEF or FEV_1 of more than 12% from baseline values strongly supports the diagnosis of asthma.[14] Some patients with asthma, however, have suboptimal responses to bronchodilator administration, and this may be related to airway edema and inflammation.[15] In these patients, a short course (1 to 3 weeks) of oral corticosteroids (20 mg PO b.i.d. in adults or 1 mg/kg/d in divided doses for children) produces significant improvement in pulmonary function if asthma exists.

Because there is considerable overlap between values of PFTs in normal and asthmatic individuals, patients with a suggestive history and 'normal' PEF or FEV_1 should also be tested for reversibility of pulmonary function after β-adrenergic agonist administration. The results of the PFTs should be evaluated using the criteria outlined above. Ninety-five percent of normal individuals have less than a 10% increase in FEV_1 after bronchodilator use.[14]

If peak flow measurements are used in the office instead of spirometry, it is strongly recommended that every patient with suspected asthma be referred for more complete pulmonary function testing at least once, to exclude other respiratory disorders that can mimic asthma. Once the diagnosis of asthma has been established, it is then reasonable to follow PEF as a longitudinal indicator of pulmonary function.[1]

Chest radiographs are not often helpful in the evaluation or management of acute exacerbations of asthma.[1,16] Indications for a chest film include asthma presenting in a very young child or a high clinical suspicion of pneumonia, pneumothorax, pneumomediastinum, or foreign-body aspiration. Allergy skin tests or a radioallergosorbent test (RAST) is also recommended in the initial evaluation of asthma because most children and more than half of adults with asthma are sensitized to respiratory allergens, and control of environmental allergens can improve asthma control.[17,18] Food allergies, however, are rarely implicated as the cause of asthma in the absence of skin or gastrointestinal symptoms.[19]

Additional studies may be indicated in selected patients. These studies may include sinus radiographs or rhinoscopies to rule out chronic sinusitis, esophageal pH monitoring to detect gastroesophageal reflux, or direct visualization of the larynx to diagnose vocal cord paralysis or dysfunction. Patients with equivocal clinical data or with incomplete responses to standard asthma therapy should be referred to an asthma specialist for additional evaluation.

Asthma Management

The goals of asthma management include restoring normal levels of activity and pulmonary function, preventing acute and chronic asthma symptoms, and avoiding adverse effects from asthma medication.[1,2] To accomplish these goals, guidelines for asthma management have been developed,[1,2] based on the current paradigm of asthma pathogenesis as a chronic inflammatory disease (Figure 1). Once the diagnosis of asthma is established, therapy should include several different components, including control of environmental triggers of asthma, use of medications to control acute and chronic airway obstruction, bronchodilators, and, importantly, patient education (Figure 1). Nonpharmacologic therapy includes modification of the environment to minimize exposure to allergens or irritants such as tobacco smoke. These recommendations are simple in theory and have proven efficacy, but, unfortunately, they may be difficult to implement. Asthma pharmacotherapy includes asthma *controllers* to treat chronic inflammation and airway obstruction and asthma *relievers* to treat acute symptoms. Patient education plays a major role in providing patients with the motivation and knowledge to achieve this goal and enhances compliance with prescribed medical therapies.[20]

The frequency and severity of asthma symptoms can be used as guides to prescribe asthma medication (Figure 3 and Tables 4 to 6).[1,2] Many patients have intermittent asthma, characterized by infrequent daytime ($\leq$2 days/wk) and nighttime ($\leq$2 nights/mo) symptoms and normal activity and pulmonary function between episodes of asthma. For these patients, an inhaled β_2-adrenergic agonist, such as albuterol (Proventil®, Ventolin®), levalbuterol (Xopenex®), or pirbuterol (Maxair™), can be used up to twice weekly as needed to relieve episodic symptoms and before strenuous activity to prevent exercise-induced bronchospasm. Nedocromil (Tilade®) or cromolyn (Intal®) are alternative preventive treatments for exercise-induced asthma.

Figure 3: Stepwise Approach for Managing Asthma in Adults and Children Older Than 5 Years[2]

Classify Severity: Clinical Features Before Treatment or Adequate Control	Symptoms/Day Symptoms/Night	PEF or FEV_1 PEF Variability
Step 4 **Severe persistent**	Continual Frequent	≤60% >30%
Step 3 **Moderate persistent**	Daily >1 night/week	>60% to <80% >30%

Notes:
- The stepwise approach is meant to assist, not replace, the clinical decision making required to meet individual patient needs.
- Classify severity: assign patient to most severe step in which any feature occurs (PEF is % of personal best; FEV_1 is % predicted).
- Gain control as quickly as possible (consider a short course of systemic corticosteroids); then step down to the least medication necessary to maintain control.

Medications Required to Maintain Long-term Control

Daily Medications

- Preferred treatment:
- High-dose inhaled corticosteroids

  and
- Long-acting β_2-agonists

  and, if needed,
- Corticosteroid tablets or syrup long term (2 mg/kg/day, generally do not exceed 60 mg/day). (Make repeat attempts to reduce systemic corticosteroids and maintain control with high-dose inhaled corticosteroids.)

- Preferred treatment:
- Low- to medium-dose inhaled corticosteroids and long-acting inhaled β_2-agonists.

- Alternative treatment
- Increase inhaled corticosteroids within medium-dose range

  or
- Low- to medium-dose inhaled corticosteroids and either leukotriene modifier or theophylline.

If needed (particularly in patients with recurring severe exacerbations):
- Preferred treatment:
- Increase inhaled corticosteroids within medium-dose range and add long-acting inhaled β_2-agonists.

- Alternative treatment:
- Increase inhaled corticosteroids within medium-dose range and add either leukotriene modifier or theophylline.

- Provide education on self-management and controlling environmental factors that make asthma worse (eg, allergens and irritants).
- Refer to an asthma specialist if there are difficulties controlling asthma or if step 4 care is required. Referral may be considered if step 3 care is required.

PEF = peak expiratory flow, FEV_1 = forced expiratory volume in 1 second

continued on next page

Figure 3: Stepwise Approach for Managing Asthma in Adults and Children Older Than 5 Years[2] *(continued)*

Classify Severity: Clinical Features Before Treatment or Adequate Control

	Symptoms/Day Symptoms/Night	PEF or FEV$_1$ PEF Variability
Step 2 Mild persistent	>2/week but <1x/day >2 nights/month	≥80% 20% to 30%
Step 1 Mild intermittent	≤2 days/week ≤2 nights/month	≥80% <20%
Quick Relief **All Patients**	■ Short-acting bronchodilator: 2 to 4 puffs short-acting inhaled β$_2$-agonists as needed for symptoms. ■ Intensity of treatment will depend on severity of exacerbation; up to three treatments at 20-minute intervals or a single nebulizer treatment as needed. Course of systemic corticosteroids may be needed. ■ Use of short-acting β$_2$-agonists >2 times a week in intermittent asthma (daily, or increasing use in persistent asthma) may indicate the need to initiate (increase) long-term control therapy.	

PEF = peak expiratory flow, FEV$_1$ = forced expiratory volume in 1 second

In contrast to intermittent asthma, patients with mild persistent asthma have symptoms that occur more than twice weekly but less than daily, and these symptoms may occasionally disturb sleep or interfere with daytime activity. Although PFTs may be within the normal range between exacerbations, studies using bronchoscopy have revealed that persistent asthma symptoms, even when mild, are usually accompanied by lower airway inflammation. Consequently, daily preventive medications, such as low-dose inhaled corticosteroids, leukotriene modifiers, cromolyn, nedocromil, or

Medications Required to Maintain Long-term Control

Daily Medications

- Preferred treatment:
- Low-dose inhaled corticosteroids.

■ Alternative treatment (listed alphabetically): cromolyn, leukotriene modifier, nedocromil, *or* sustained-release theophylline to serum concentrations of 5 to 15 µg/mL.

■ No daily medication needed.

■ Severe exacerbations may occur, separated by long periods of normal lung function and no symptoms. A course of systemic corticosteroids is recommended.

Step down:
Review treatment every 1 to 6 months; a gradual stepwise reduction in treatment may be possible.

Step up:
If control is not maintained, consider step up. First, review patient medication technique, adherence, and environmental control.

oral theophylline, are now recommended to control mild persistent asthma. Inhaled corticosteroids are the most potent and effective anti-inflammatory medications. In children, cromolyn sodium and leukotriene receptor antagonists are alternative therapies for mild, persistent asthma because of their excellent safety records,[21,22] while inhaled corticosteroids (Table 6) are preferred for adolescents and adults because they are generally more effective.[23] The leukotriene receptor antagonists (zafirlukast [Accolate®], montelukast [Singulair®]) and synthesis inhibitors (zileuton [Zyflo®])

Table 4: Usual Dosages for Quick-Relief Medications*

Medication	Dosage form	Adult dose
Short-Acting Inhaled β-Agonists		
	Metered-dose inhaler	
albuterol albuterol HFA	90 μg/puff, 200 puffs	2 puffs 5 min before exercise or 2 puffs t.i.d.-q.i.d. p.r.n.
bitolterol	370 μg/puff, 300 puffs	
pirbuterol	200 μg/puff, 400 puffs	
terbutaline	200 μg/puff, 300 puffs	
	Dry powder inhaler	
albuterol Rotahaler®	200 μg/capsule	1-2 capsules q 4-6 h as needed, or before exercise
	Nebulizer solution	
albuterol	5 mg/mL (0.5%)	1.25-5.0 mg (0.25-1 cc) in 2-3 cc of saline q 4-8 h
	0.083% (unit dose vials)	3 mL (2.5 mg) q 4-8 h
levalbuterol	0.63 mg or 1.25 mg vials	0.63-1.25 mg q 6-8 h
Systemic Corticosteroids		
methylpred-nisolone	2-, 4-, 8-, 16-, 32-mg tablets	Short course 'burst': 40-60 mg/d as single or 2 divided doses for 3-10 days
prednisolone	5-mg tabs, 5 mg/tsp, 15 mg/tsp	Same as for methylprednisolone
prednisone	1-, 2-, 5-, 10-, 20-, 25-mg tabs; 5 mg/tsp	Same as for methylprednisolone

*Modified from reference 1.

Child dose	Comments
1-2 puffs 5 min before exercise	An increasing use or lack of expected effect indicates diminished control of asthma.
	or
2 puffs t.i.d.-q.i.d. p.r.n.	Not generally recommended for long-term treatment. Daily regular use indicates the need for additional long-term control therapy.
	Differences in potency exist so that all products are essentially equipotent on a per-puff basis.
	May double usual dose for mild exacerbations.
	Nonselective agents (ie, epinephrine, isoproterenol, metaproterenol) are not recommended.
1 capsule q 4-6 h as needed before exercise	
0.05 mg/kg (min 1.25 mg, max 2.5 mg) in 2-3 cc of saline q 4-6 h	May mix with cromolyn or ipratropium nebulizer solutions. May double dose for mild exacerbations.
0.1 mL/kg (min 1.5 mL, max 3.0 mL) q 4-6 h	
0.31-0.63 mg neb q 6-8 h	May be useful in patients in whom albuterol is effective, but causes significant side effects.
Short course 'burst': 1-2 mg/kg/d, maximum 60 mg/d, for 3-10 days	Short courses of 'bursts' are effective for establishing control when initiating therapy or during a period of gradual deterioration. The burst should be continued until patient achieves 80% personal best peak expiratory flow or symptoms resolve. This usually requires 3-10 days but may require longer. There is no evidence that tapering the dose after improvement prevents relapse.
Same as for methylprednisolone	
Same as for methylprednisolone	

Table 5: Usual Dosages for Long-term Control Medications[2]

Medication	Dosage form
Inhaled Corticosteroids *(see Table 6)*	
Systemic Corticosteroids *(Applies to all three corticosteroids)*	
methylprednisolone	2-, 4-, 8-, 16-, 32-mg tablets
prednisolone	5-mg tablets, 5 mg/5 cc, 15 mg/5 cc
prednisone	1-, 2.5-, 5-, 10-, 20-, 50-mg tablets; 5 mg/cc, 5 mg/5 cc
Long-acting Inhaled β$_2$-agonists *(Should not be used for symptom relief or for exacerbations. Use with inhaled corticosteroids.)*	
salmeterol	MDI 21 µg/puff DPI 50 µg/blister
formoterol	DPI 12 µg/single-use capsule
Combined Medication	
fluticasone/salmeterol	DPI 100, 250, or 500 µg/50 µg
Cromolyn and Nedocromil	
cromolyn	MDI 1 mg/puff Nebulizer 20 mg/ampule
nedocromil	MDI 1.75 mg/puff

MDI = metered-dose inhaler, DPI = dry powder inhaler

Adult dose	Child dose (≤12 yr of age)
• 7.5 to 60 mg/d in a single dose in AM or q.o.d. as needed for control • Short-course 'burst' to achieve control: 40 to 60 mg/d as single or 2 divided doses for 3 to 10 d	• 0.25 to 2 mg/kg/d in a single dose in AM or q.o.d. as needed for control • Short-course 'burst': 1 to 2 mg/kg/d, maximum 60 mg/d for 3 to 10 d
2 puffs q 12 h 1 blister q 12 h 1 capsule q 12 h	1 to 2 puffs q 12 h 1 blister q 12 h 1 capsule q 12 h
1 inhalation b.i.d.; dose depends on severity of asthma	1 inhalation b.i.d.; dose depends on severity of asthma
2 to 4 puffs t.i.d. to q.i.d. 1 ampule t.i.d. to q.i.d. 2 to 4 puffs b.i.d. to q.i.d.	1 to 2 puffs t.i.d. to q.i.d. 1 ampule t.i.d. to q.i.d. 1 to 2 puffs b.i.d. to q.i.d.

continued on next page

Table 5: Usual Dosages for Long-term Control Medications[2]
(continued)

Medication	Dosage form
Leukotriene Modifiers	
montelukast	4- or 5-mg chewable tablet, 10-mg tablet
zafirlukast	10- or 20-mg tablet
zileuton	300- or 600-mg tablet
Methylxanthines *(Serum monitoring is important [serum concentration of 5 to 15 µg/mL at steady state].)*	
theophylline	Liquids, sustained-release tablets, and capsules

MDI = metered-dose inhaler, DPI = dry powder inhaler

constitute a new class of medications that produce long-lasting bronchodilation and reduce blood eosinophil counts and antigen-induced eosinophil recruitment.[24] These properties suggest that these new medications may be useful in the long-term control of mild persistent asthma. In addition to controller medications, inhaled β_2-adrenergic agonists may be used up to four times daily to relieve acute symptoms. Chronic overuse of a β_2-adrenergic agonist may indicate continued inflammation in the lower airway, signaling the need to reevaluate asthma triggers and the preventive medication regimen.

Adult dose	Child dose (≤12 yr of age)
10 mg qhs	4 mg qhs (2 to 5 yr)
	5 mg qhs (6 to 14 yr)
	10 mg qhs (>14 yr)
40 mg daily	20 mg daily (5 to 11 yr)
(20-mg tablet b.i.d.)	(10-mg tablet b.i.d.)
2,400 mg daily	
(give tablets q.i.d.)	

Starting dose 10 mg/kg/d up to 300 mg max; usual max 800 mg/d	Starting dose 10 mg/kg/d; usual max: • <1 yr of age: 0.2 (age in weeks) + 5 = mg/kg/d • ≥1 yr of age: 16 mg/kg/d

Moderately severe asthma is usually accompanied by daily symptoms (before treatment is initiated), disturbance of sleep or daytime activities more than once weekly, and, occasionally, more severe exacerbations requiring acute care visits to the doctor's office or hospital emergency room. Pulmonary function tests often show signs of airway obstruction, at least before anti-inflammatory therapy has been instituted. For moderate asthma, the preferred therapy consists of low- to medium-dose inhaled corticosteroid combined with a long-acting inhaled β-agonist. This approach provides improved symptom relief,

Table 6: Estimated Comparative Daily Dosages for Inhaled Corticosteroids[2]

Drug	Low daily dose	
	Adult	**Child***
beclomethasone CFC 42 or 84 µg/puff	168 to 504 µg	84 to 336 µg
beclomethasone HFA 40 or 80 µg/puff	80 to 240 µg	80 to 160 µg
budesonide DPI 200 µg/inhalation	200 to 600 µg	200 to 400 µg
budesonide inhalation suspension for nebulization (child dose)		0.5 mg
flunisolide 250 µg/puff	500 to 1,000 µg	500 to 750 µg
fluticasone MDI: 44, 110, or 220 µg/puff	88 to 264 µg	88 to 176 µg
DPI: 50, 100, or 250 µg/inhalation	100 to 300 µg	100 to 200 µg
triamcinolone acetonide 100 µg/puff	400 to 1,000 µg	400 to 800 µg

* Children ≤12 years of age

lung function, and protection from asthma exacerbations compared to higher doses of an inhaled corticosteroid alone.[25,26] The leukotriene modifiers or theophylline can also be used as an adjunct to inhaled corticosteroids in patients with moderate asthma.

Medium daily dose		High daily dose	
Adult	Child*	Adult	Child*
504 to 840 µg	336 to 672 µg	>840 µg	>672 µg
240 to 480 µg	160 to 320 µg	>480 µg	>320 µg
600 to 1,200 µg	400 to 800 µg	>1,200 µg	>800 µg
	1.0 mg		2.0 mg
1,000 to 2,000 µg	1,000 to 1,250 µg	>2,000 µg	>1,250 µg
264 to 660 µg	176 to 440 µg	>660 µg	>440 µg
300 to 600 µg	200 to 400 µg	>600 µg	>400 µg
1,000 to 2,000 µg	800 to 1,200 µg	>2,000 µg	>1,200 µg

It is especially important to identify patients who have severe asthma so that aggressive intervention can prevent serious morbidity or even fatal attacks. Severe asthma is usually accompanied by daily wheezing and frequent exacerbations. These patients typically have a history of frequent visits to emergency rooms or acute outpatient visits for asthma. Hospitalization is common in this group, and the occurrence of respiratory failure with intubation should be a 'red flag' for the identification of patients at increased risk for additional severe asthma exacerbations. These patients typically have poor exercise tolerance that limits their physical activities, and they experience frequent night awakening. Pulmonary function tests reveal significant airway obstruction that often does not completely reverse with bronchodilator use. Medical therapy is more intensive for these patients and often includes high-dose inhaled corticosteroids, which may be supplemented by daily or every-other-day oral corticosteroids. Adjunctive therapy to provide greater control of symptoms and miminize the required dose of oral corticosteroid may include long-acting β_2-agonists, sustained-release theophylline, and a leukotriene receptor antagonist or synthesis inhibitor.[1,2,24]

Compliance with medical therapy should be carefully assessed in patients with moderate to severe asthma because poor control of asthma can signal underuse of asthma controller medications.[1] Unfortunately, estimating compliance is difficult. There is no correlation between compliance and income, gender, ethnicity, or physician assessment. However, several measures are helpful in estimating and improving compliance. First, the physician can call the pharmacist to determine if prescriptions are being filled or look at the date printed on the patient's medication container. Second, the physician can find out how the patient perceives the prescribed medications, especially in terms of side effects, efficacy, cost, and 'steroid phobia.' Finally, the physician should make the regimen as simple as possible and always provide a written treatment plan (Table 7) so that the patient has a clear understanding of the prescribed therapy. Many fine educational materials can be obtained from the National Asthma Education and Prevention Program (NAEPP, PO Box 30105, Bethesda, MD 20824-0105; telephone 301-951-3260; Web site http://www.nhlbi.nih.gov/about/naepp).

The recent trend toward reliance on inhaled medication for treating asthma is well supported by data proving the efficacy and relative safety of these products. However, improper use of an MDI is a common problem leading to suboptimal responses to asthma treatment regimens. Technique should always be reviewed with the patient after prescribing an inhaled medication (Table 8), and it is most helpful to have the patient demonstrate his or her inhaler technique at each outpatient visit. Spacer devices (Aerochamber®, Inspirease®, and others) can increase inhaler effectiveness and reduce side effects, especially in patients with suboptimal inhaler technique.[27] Selection of the spacer is determined by many factors, including the age of the patient, the type of MDI or medication, and the cost. Use of a spacer device with an inhaler does not eliminate the need to carefully review proper administration technique with the patient or parent, preferably during the clinic visit.

Monitoring of pulmonary function at home with a peak flow meter can increase awareness of asthma and encourage self-management skills by providing a guide for administration of bronchodilators.[1] Peak flow meters provide a reasonably accurate and portable means of obtaining objective pulmonary function measurements. These devices measure PEF, which is the greatest flow velocity (L/min) that is generated during forced expiration. This measurement correlates well with FEV_1, and these values, when combined with clinical information such as symptoms and medication requirements, can be used by the patient, parent, and physician to make intelligent decisions about asthma therapy. Use of a peak flow meter may also have psychologic benefits for children and adolescents by allowing them to effectively manage most asthmatic exacerbations and by providing positive feedback for the asthma treatment plan, thereby increasing feelings of self-control over their chronic disease. In addition, peak flow meters may be useful in evaluating the possibility of asthma in a patient who has suggestive symptoms at night or after exercise, yet

Table 7: Suggested Content for a Written Asthma Control Plan

- Instructions to control exposure to environmental allergens and irritants

- Guidelines for monitoring peak expiratory flow:
  - Establish personal best value
  - Establish green, yellow, and red zones

- Provide written instructions regarding medication use:
  - Maintenance medications
  - Prophylaxis for exercise, allergen exposure, etc.
  - Rescue medications

- Provide contact telephone numbers to report acute asthma symptoms:
  - Clinic
  - Emergency services

has normal pulmonary function at the time of evaluation. It should be emphasized that PEF readings, especially those obtained at home, should be interpreted with an understanding that there are many causes of falsely low or high readings, such as malfunction of the instrument, errors in technique, or manipulation of the data for secondary gain.

A useful protocol for using peak flow meters in managing asthma is outlined in the *Guidelines for the Diagnosis and Management of Asthma,* published by the U.S. Department of Health and Human Services.[1] The first goal is to ascertain the patient's personal best peak flow rate, which requires the appropriate use of medications to maximize pulmonary function. Once this value has been established, the calculation of green (80% to 100% of personal best), yellow (50% to 80% of personal best), and red (<50% of personal best) zones can be accomplished. Peak flow rates in the green zone indicate stable disease activity, provided

Table 8: Proper Inhaler Technique*

- Remove cap and hold inhaler upright.
- Shake the inhaler.
- Tilt head back slightly and breathe out.
- Use a spacer device, or open mouth** and place inhaler 1-2 inches away.
- Press down on inhaler to release medication as you start to breathe in slowly.
- Breathe in slowly (over 3-5 seconds) and hold breath for 5-10 seconds.
- Repeat puffs as directed. Wait 1 minute between puffs.

* Adapted from NAEPP guidelines.[1] Spacer devices are especially recommended for children and the elderly. For dry powder inhalers, see package insert.

**For breath-activated inhalers, the inhaler opening must be held in the mouth with lips closed.

no other warning signs are present (eg, nocturnal awakenings due to asthma, exercise intolerance). If the peak flow rate is in the yellow zone and administration of a β-agonist does not bring it back into the green zone, many asthma specialists would recommend increasing (double or higher) the maintenance dose of inhaled corticosteroid until peak flow rates are consistently back in the green zone.[28] If peak flow rates continue to deteriorate while in the yellow zone or are in the red zone, oral corticosteroid therapy (prednisone 20 mg PO b.i.d. or 0.5 to 1 mg/kg/d for children, administered for 5 to 10 days) should be initiated, and the patient should contact a physician as soon as possible. Although prednisone given over short periods has relatively few side effects, extra caution must be used in prescribing oral corticosteroid therapy to patients with significant health problems such as diabetes, hypertension, or glaucoma. In addition, patients who develop varicella within 30 days of receiving a course of oral corticosteroids may require specific antiviral therapy, although patients receiving standard doses of inhaled corticosteroids do not appear to be at increased risk.[29]

Summary

Accurate diagnosis of asthma requires the use of objective measurement of pulmonary function in addition to careful evaluation of history and physical findings. Treatment should be tailored to the individual patient, based on identification of triggers for acute symptoms and classification of disease severity. Optimal control of asthma symptoms is achieved using a combination of patient education, environmental modifications, and medical therapy, which should include topical anti-inflammatory drugs for all but mild disease. Goals of therapy include restoring normal pulmonary function and controlling symptoms while avoiding side effects from asthma medications.

References

1. National Asthma Education and Prevention Program, National Heart, Lung, and Blood Institute, National Institutes of Health: Expert Panel Report II: *Guidelines for the Diagnosis and Management of Asthma*. Bethesda, U.S. Department of Health and Human Services, 1997.

2. National Asthma Education and Prevention Program, National Heart, Lung, and Blood Institute: *Guidelines for the Diagnosis and Management of Asthma—Update on Selected Topics 2002*. NIH Publication No. 02-5075, July 2002.

3. Warner A, Boushey HA, Lee TH, et al, eds: The genetics of asthma. *Am J Respir Crit Care Med* 1997;156:S67-S156.

4. Busse WW, Lemanske RF Jr: Asthma. *N Engl J Med* 2001; 344:350-362.

5. Colasurdo GN, Larsen GL: Airway hyperresponsiveness. In: Busse WW, Holgate ST, eds. *Asthma and Rhinitis*. Boston, Blackwell Scientific Publications, 1995, pp 1044-1056.

6. Gern JE, Busse WW: The role of viral infections in the natural history of asthma. *J Allergy Clin Immunol* 2000;106:201-212.

7. Reed CE: The natural history of asthma in adults: the problem of irreversibility. *J Allergy Clin Immunol* 1999;103:539-547.

8. Litonjua AA, Carey VJ, Burge HA, et al: Parental history and the risk for childhood asthma. Does mother confer more risk than father? *Am J Respir Crit Care Med* 1998;158:176-181.

9. Bloomberg GR, Strunk RC: Crisis in asthma care. *Pediatr Clin North Am* 1992;39:1225-1241.

10. O'Hollaren MT, Yunginger JW, Offord KP, et al: Exposure to an aeroallergen as a possible precipitating factor in respiratory arrest in young patients with asthma. *N Engl J Med* 1991;324:359-363.

11. Shim CS, Williams MH Jr: Relationship of wheezing to the severity of obstruction in asthma. *Arch Intern Med* 1983;143:890-892.

12. Bush RK, Asbury D: Aspirin-sensitive asthma. In: Busse WW, Holgate ST, eds. *Asthma and Rhinitis*. Boston, Blackwell Scientific Publications, 1995, pp 1429-1439.

13. Stern RC, Boat TF, Wood RE, et al: Treatment and prognosis of nasal polyps in cystic fibrosis. *Am J Dis Child* 1982;136:1067-1070.

14. American Thoracic Society: Lung function testing: selection of reference values and interpretative strategies. *Am Rev Respir Dis* 1991;144:1202-1218.

15. Enright PL, Lebowitz MD, Cockroft DW: Physiologic measures: pulmonary function tests. Asthma outcome. *Am J Respir Crit Care Med* 1994;149:S9-S18-S22.

16. Gershel JC, Goldman HS, Stein RE, et al: The usefulness of chest radiographs in first asthma attacks. *N Engl J Med* 1983;309:336-339.

17. Bush RK, Gern JE: Allergy evaluation: who, what and how. In: Schidlow DV, Smith DS, eds. *A Practical Guide to Pediatric Respiratory Diseases*. Philadelphia, Hanley & Belfus, 1994, pp 261-270.

18. Ingram JM, Heymann PW: Environmental controls in the management of asthma. *Immunol Allergy Clin North Am* 1993;13:785-801.

19. James JM, Bernhisel-Broadbent J, Sampson HA: Respiratory reactions provoked by double-blind food challenges in children. *Am J Respir Crit Care Med* 1994;149:59-64.

20. National Asthma Education and Prevention Program, National Heart, Lung, and Blood Institute, National Institutes of Health: *Teach Your Patients About Asthma: A Clinician's Guide*. Bethesda, U.S. Department of Health and Human Services, 1992.

21. Murphy S: Cromolyn sodium: basic mechanisms and clinical usage. *Pediatr Allergy Immunol* 1988;2:237-254.

22. Graham LM: Balancing safety and efficacy in the treatment of pediatric asthma. *J Allergy Clin Immunol* 2002;109:S560-S566.

23. Barnes PJ: Inhaled corticosteroids for asthma. *N Engl J Med* 1993;332:868-874.

24. Bisgaard H: Pathophysiology of the cystinyl leukotrienes and effects of leukotriene receptor antagonists in asthma. *Allergy* 2001;(suppl 66):7-11.

25. Zetterstrom O, Buhl R, Mellem H, et al: Improved asthma control with budesonide/formoterol in a single inhaler, compared with budesonide alone. *Eur Respir J* 2001;18:262-268.

26. Markham A, Jarvis B: Inhaled salmeterol/fluticasone propionate combination: a review of its use in persistent asthma. *Drugs* 2000;60:1207-1233.

27. McFadden ER Jr: Improper patient techniques with metered dose inhalers: clinical consequences and solutions to misuse. *J Allergy Clin Immunol* 1995;96:278-283.

28. Volovitz B, et al: Effectiveness and safety of inhaled corticosteroids in controlling acute asthma attacks in children who were treated in the emergency department: a controlled comparative study with oral prednisolone. *J Allergy Clin Immunol* 1998;102:605-609.

29. Executive Committee, American Academy of Allergy and Immunology: Inhaled corticosteroids and severe viral infections. *J Allergy Clin Immunol* 1993;92:223-228.

8

Management of Acute Asthma Exacerbations

A sthma is a chronic inflammatory disease of the airways characterized by episodic airway obstruction of variable duration and intensity. Many asthma attacks can be controlled by the use of rescue medicine such as inhaled β_2-adrenergic agonists or bursts of oral prednisone (Deltasone®). However, symptoms sometimes progressively worsen over minutes, hours, or days despite the use of inhaled or oral bronchodilators. At the far end of the spectrum is status asthmaticus, which is defined as unremitting asthma symptoms that put the patient at risk for respiratory failure.

The most effective strategy for dealing with status asthmaticus is prevention, achieved by recognition of the first signs and symptoms of progressively worsening asthma and by the early use of oral or high-dose inhaled corticosteroids. This chapter outlines the office or emergency room management of patients who have not received, or have not responded favorably to, early interventions and have proceeded to develop acute severe exacerbations of asthma.

Clinical Assessment

Patients with severe asthma symptoms should be evaluated quickly. In fact, it is best to begin treatment even while the evaluation is in progress. Of course, patients with severe dyspnea should not be left to sit in a reception area unattended. Therefore, personnel working in the reception area must be trained to triage patients with severe asthma episodes directly into a treatment area.

A patient's medical history provides important clues about the severity of the episode. It is essential to obtain a complete description of the factors that trigger asthma symptoms, of the risk factors for severe asthma exacerbations, and of the asthma medications being used. This information guides immediate therapy and can be helpful later in determining the disposition of patients who experience only partial improvement after emergency room therapy.[1-4] Medical history features that indicate a high risk for asthma-associated morbidity and mortality include previous intubation or intensive care unit (ICU) admission, poor compliance with prescribed medical therapy, underappreciation of asthma symptoms, psychiatric conditions, *Alternaria* allergy, or hospitalization despite the chronic use of oral corticosteroids.[1,2,5] Asthma that has been building in severity over several days may be particularly difficult to reverse in the emergency room. These high-risk patients require extra attention, including intensive efforts at patient education directed at preventing future episodes of severe asthma. The patient's treatment regimen should be carefully assessed. Excessive bronchodilator use is an important indicator of asthma disease severity, and underuse of preventive medications such as inhaled corticosteroids is often a factor in poorly controlled asthma.

Useful indicators of asthma severity on physical examination include the respiratory rate, the degree of respiratory distress, the use of accessory muscles of respiration, the presence or absence of wheezing, and the degree of air movement with respiration.[1-4] The patient's general appearance can be diagnostically important. Cyanosis or impaired consciousness are obvious signs of impending respiratory failure, but restlessness, somnolence, fatigue, and inability to recline are also signs of severe respiratory compromise.

The pulsus paradoxus, which is the difference between systolic blood pressures measured during inspiration and expiration, correlates closely with the level of airway obstruction. A pulsus paradoxus of greater than 10 to 15 mm Hg indicates severe respiratory distress.[4]

Because symptoms and physical findings are not always reliable indicators of the degree of airway obstruction,[6,7] objective measurements of pulmonary function have paramount importance in the management of acute asthma. Spirometry is particularly helpful in detecting small-airway obstruction and in detecting conditions, such as vocal cord dysfunction, that can mimic asthma. Useful indices include forced expiratory volume in 1 second (FEV_1), the ratio of FEV_1 to forced vital capacity (FEV_1/FVC), and midexpiratory forced expiratory flow (FEF_{25-75}).[8] If a spirometer is not available in the emergency room, a peak expiratory flow meter can also provide useful information. Patient values for pulmonary function tests should be compared to the patient's personal best, if this is known, or to standardized norms.[8] Objective measurements of pulmonary function are also used to measure the response to bronchodilator therapy. In conjunction with trends in symptoms and physical findings, these measurements are used to guide the immediate treatment of acute asthma, and they influence decisions regarding hospitalization (Figure 1).

Measurement of arterial blood gases or oxygen saturation by pulse oximetry adds little to the management of mild asthma, but is indicated for patients who present with moderate or severe airway obstruction. Hypoxia is common once pulmonary function measurements such as FEV_1 or peak expiratory flow (PEF) are less than 50% of predicted.[9] Hypercapnia occurs most often in patients whose FEV_1 is less than 25% of predicted.

Therapy for Status Asthmaticus

Patients who present with severe respiratory distress must receive immediate therapy (Figure 1). A quick assessment of

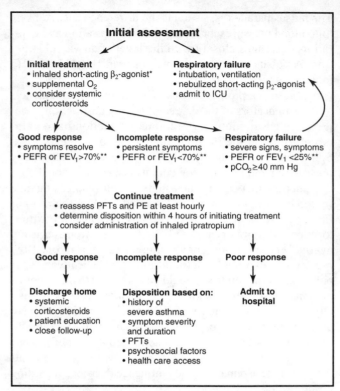

Figure 1: Treatment of status asthmaticus. *Use a rapid-onset β$_2$-adrenergic agonist such as albuterol via either nebulizer or MDI. Up to three doses may be given at 20-minute intervals in the first hour, and clinical status should be reassessed after each dose. **Pulmonary function tests (PFTs) should be compared to the patient's personal best or, if these data are unavailable, to published standards.[8]

respiratory status should be performed to establish baseline values and to identify patients with respiratory failure who need intensive care and possibly intubation. Nebulized β$_2$-agonists and oxygen should be administered even if preparations for intubation are taking place because responses to inhaled medication may sometimes be dramatic and obviate the need for intubation. The treatment of choice for status asthmaticus is the administration of up to three nebulized doses of a short-acting β_2-agonist (albuterol [Proventil®, Ventolin®] or levalbuterol [Xopenex®]) spaced 20 minutes apart (Table 1).[1,2,4,10] Although β_2-adrenergic agonists are used in higher than standard doses during exacerbations, serious side effects are rare.[11] Milder symptoms occur in many patients, including tremor, mild tachycardia, and nervousness. Continuous administration of albuterol may produce greater improvement than intermittent dosing in some patient groups, including children and severely affected adults.[1]

Evidence is now accumulating that metered-dose inhalers (MDIs) can be just as effective as nebulized medications in treating acute asthma.[12,13] MDIs have the advantages of delivering medications more quickly and less expensively; however, patients in severe distress may lack the coordination and breath-holding ability needed for best results.

Administration of systemic corticosteroids either orally or parenterally should be considered early in the course of status asthmaticus.[1,2,4,10] Oral corticosteroids are superior to high-dose inhaled corticosteroids for acute severe asthma because they provide greater improvements in pulmonary function and reduce the risk for hospitalization.[14] Early corticosteroid use may decrease the need for hospitalization and reduce the frequency of readmissions to the emergency suite.[14,15]

Although short-acting β_2-adrenergic agonists are the bronchodilators of choice for acute asthma, anticholinergic medications such as ipratropium (Atrovent®) may augment the effect of these medications in acute asthma.[16] Ipratropium, an atropine-like drug with minimal systemic side effects when administered topically, is now available in both an MDI and a nebulizer solution. The usual dose of ipratropium in acute asthma is 2.5 mL (0.5 mg) delivered via nebulization, or 2 to 4 puffs via MDI with a spacer device, giv-

Table 1: Medication Doses in Acute Asthma

Class	Medication	Form
β₂-agonist	albuterol (Proventil®, Ventolin®)	0.5% nebulizer solution 0.083% nebulizer solution MDI (90 µg/puff)
	levalbuterol (Xopenex®)	0.63 mg or 1.25 mg vials
Injected adrenergic agonists	epinephrine	1:1000 solution
	terbutaline	1 mg/mL solution
Anticholinergic	ipratropium (Atrovent®)	0.02% nebulizer solution MDI (18 µg/puff)
Corticosteroids	prednisone (Deltasone®)	Oral (tablets or 5 mg/5 mL syrup)
	prednisolone (Pediapred®, Prelone®)	Oral syrup (5 mg or 15 mg/5 mL)
	methylprednisolone (Solu-Medrol®)	IV solution

en 1 to 3 times at 20-minute intervals. If clinical improvement is observed, anticholinergic therapy can be continued at less frequent intervals.

Aminophylline is no longer recommended for treating acute exacerbations of asthma in the emergency department. Several studies, including a meta-analysis, have found no evidence that aminophylline is beneficial in acute asthma that has been treated with inhaled β₂-agonists and

Adult Dose	Pediatric Dose
0.5 mL neb q 20 min (dilute in 2 mL normal saline) 3 mL neb q 20 min 4-8 puffs inh q 20 min 0.63-1.25 mg neb q 6-8 h	0.25-0.5 mL neb q 20 min (dilute in 2 mL normal saline) 1.5-3 mL neb q 20 min 4-8 puffs inh q 20 min 0.31-0.63 mg neb q 6-8 h
0.3 mL sub-Q q 20 min 0.25 mL sub-Q q 20 min	0.01 mL/kg sub-Q q 20 min (maximum dose 0.3 mL) 0.01 mL/kg sub-Q q 20 min (maximum dose 0.25 mL)
2.5 mL neb q 20 min 2-4 puffs inh q 20 min	1.25-2.5 mL neb q 20 min 2 puffs inh q 20 min
60 mg PO q.d. in single or divided doses 60-80 mg IV q 6-8 h	0.5-2.0 mg/kg/d in single or divided doses (maximum 60 mg/d) 1-2 mg/kg IV q 6 h (maximum 120 mg/d)

systemic corticosteroids.[17,18] Intravenous magnesium sulfate has been evaluated for use in acute asthma, but clinical responses are inconsistent, and it cannot be recommended for routine use.[19] Finally, no data are available to support the use of leukotriene modifiers in acute asthma.

The respiratory status of patients presenting with status asthmaticus should be reassessed at frequent intervals. Many emergency departments have developed flow sheets for recording serial measurements of pulmonary function, physical findings, and oxygenation to facilitate monitoring.

Disposition

Patients who respond well to emergency therapy, with improved pulmonary function and resolved signs and symptoms of asthma, can be discharged home (Figure 1). Oral or inhaled corticosteroids may be prescribed to reduce the chance of recurrent symptoms and return visits to the emergency room.[20,21] Regardless of the medical therapy prescribed, it is important to maintain close medical follow-up either by telephone or a scheduled clinic appointment. In general, these patients should be seen within 1 week of any emergency room visit to reassess their respiratory status and to adjust maintenance therapy to minimize the chance of future exacerbations of asthma.

Patients who have an incomplete response to therapy may require continued treatment with bronchodilators and corticosteroids in the emergency room, but the disposition should be determined within 4 to 6 hours after initiating treatment. Most patients who experience partial improvement after emergency treatment may be discharged home with close medical follow-up. However, hospital admission may be the best course for patients with prolonged episodes of airway obstruction, for those with a history of previous hospital admissions (especially those associated with respiratory failure), or for those with psychosocial factors that may impede the successful treatment of asthma.[1,2]

Patients with a poor response to emergency room treatment of asthma should be admitted to the hospital to continue close observation, bronchodilator therapy, and anti-inflammatory therapy. Indications for hospital admission include hypoxia, hypercapnia, or persistent severe airway obstruction (PEF <40% of predicted).[1,2] ICU consultation should be made early for those patients at risk for respiratory failure as indicated by extreme dyspnea, poor objective measurements of pulmonary function, or hypercapnia.

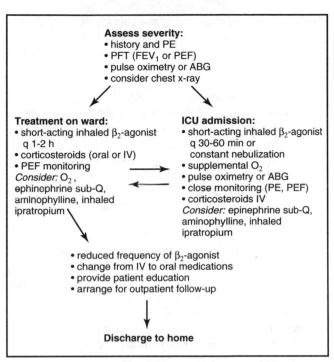

Assess severity:
• history and PE
• PFT (FEV_1 or PEF)
• pulse oximetry or ABG
• consider chest x-ray

Treatment on ward:
• short-acting inhaled β_2-agonist q 1-2 h
• corticosteroids (oral or IV)
• PEF monitoring
Consider: O_2, epinephrine sub-Q, aminophylline, inhaled ipratropium

ICU admission:
• short-acting inhaled β_2-agonist q 30-60 min or constant nebulization
• supplemental O_2
• pulse oximetry or ABG
• close monitoring (PE, PEF)
• corticosteroids IV
Consider: epinephrine sub-Q, aminophylline, inhaled ipratropium

• reduced frequency of β_2-agonist
• change from IV to oral medications
• provide patient education
• arrange for outpatient follow-up

Discharge to home

Figure 2: Hospital management of asthma. PFT = pulmonary function test; PE = physical examination; PEF = peak expiratory flow; ABG = arterial blood gas.

We recommend that all patients be observed for at least 30 minutes after their last dose of β_2-agonist to ensure that they are stable before being discharged from the emergency room. All patients discharged from the emergency room should be given a written asthma treatment plan and contingency instructions to be followed if their symptoms worsen.

Hospital Therapy of Asthma

Cooperation and communication between the emergency room or clinic and the inpatient ward are crucial to ensure uninterrupted monitoring and therapy (Figure 2). Because lung function is intrinsically unstable during an asthma attack, severe respiratory distress can develop even in patients who appear to be improving. Pulmonary function before and after β_2-agonist therapy should be serially monitored in the hospital with a bedside peak flow meter.[1,22] Monitoring of oxygenation with pulse oximetry or arterial blood gases may be required in patients with more severe disease. Chest radiograph should be considered for patients with severe dyspnea or unequal breath sounds, but radiographs contribute little to the management of patients in the absence of these findings.[4]

Inpatient medical therapy should include administration of short-acting inhaled β_2-agonists every 1 to 2 hours.[11] Inhaled ipratropium can also be added if there is an inadequate response to β_2-agonist alone. Oral or intravenous corticosteroids should be used to treat underlying airway inflammation. Intravenous aminophylline can be considered as an adjunct bronchodilator, but as is the case with use of this drug in the emergency room, its benefits have not been universally demonstrated in controlled studies.[17,19] Oxygen should be given to hypoxic patients and to those with unstable pulmonary function.

ICU admission is required for patients who are at risk for respiratory failure, as indicated by clinical evidence of fatigue or progressively worsening dyspnea, FEV_1 or PEF less than 30% of predicted, or hypercapnia.[1,2] Short-acting β_2-adrenergic agonists should be administered every 30 to 60 minutes or by constant nebulization. Patients on high doses of β_2-adrenergic agonists should have cardiac monitoring to detect cardiac arrhythmias. Occasionally, airway obstruction that is resistant to inhaled β_2-adrenergic agonists responds to either nebulized ipratropium or subcutaneous epinephrine.[23,24] Corticosteroids should generally be administered intravenously every 6 to 8 hours. The decision to intubate and mechanically ventilate is usually based on clinical evidence of progressive respiratory distress and impending respiratory failure, rather than on any set criteria for pulmonary function or arterial blood gas results.

Once a patient is improving, the frequency of inhaled medication can be reduced, and medications that are being delivered intravenously should be changed to oral preparations. Efforts at patient education should begin as soon as this is practical. That education should focus on identifying asthma triggers and the appropriate use of anti-inflammatory and bronchodilator medications.[25] Oral corticosteroids should be prescribed, with a schedule that tapers to zero (or maintenance requirements) within 1 to 2 weeks of discharge. A follow-up outpatient visit should be arranged before the patient leaves the hospital.

Summary

Acute severe asthma is a medical emergency, and, as with all emergencies, successful outcome depends on the prompt recognition of signs and symptoms, leading to the initiation of appropriate therapy. Every effort should be made to ensure that patients with frequent emergency room visits follow up with their regular health-care provider or an asthma specialist so that maintenance regimens can be designed to minimize the chances of future exacerbations of asthma.

References

1. National Asthma Education and Prevention Program, National Heart, Lung, and Blood Institute, National Institutes of Health: Expert Panel Report II: *Guidelines for the Diagnosis and Management of Asthma.* Bethesda, U.S. Department of Health and Human Services, 1997.

2. *Global Initiative for Asthma: Global Strategy for Asthma Management and Prevention.* NHLBI/WHO Workshop Report, Publication No: 95-3659. Bethesda, MD, National Institutes of Health, 1995.

3. American Thoracic Society: Standards for the diagnosis and care of patients with chronic obstructive pulmonary disease (COPD) and asthma. *Am Rev Respir Dis* 1987;136:225-244.

4. Corbridge TC, Hall JB: The assessment and management of adults with status asthmaticus. *Am J Respir Crit Care Med* 1995; 151:1296-1316.

5. O'Hollaren MT, Yunginger JW, Offord KP, et al: Exposure to an aeroallergen as a possible precipitating factor in respiratory arrest in young patients with asthma. *N Engl J Med* 1991;324: 359-363.

6. McFadden ER Jr, Kiser R, DeGroot WJ: Acute bronchial asthma: relations between clinical and physiologic manifestations. *N Engl J Med* 1973;288:221-225.

7. Shim CS, Williams MH Jr: Relationship of wheezing to the severity of obstruction in asthma. *Arch Intern Med* 1983; 143:890-892.

8. American Thoracic Society: Lung function testing: selection of reference values and interpretative strategies. *Am Rev Respir Dis* 1991;144:1202-1218.

9. Nowak RM, Tomlanovich MC, Sarkar DD, et al: Arterial blood gases and pulmonary function testing in acute bronchial asthma. Predicting patient outcomes. *JAMA* 1983;249:2043-2046.

10. Provisional Committee on Quality Improvement, American Academy of Pediatrics: Practice parameter: the office management of acute exacerbations of asthma in children. *Pediatrics* 1994;93:119-126.

11. Gern JE, Lemanske RF: Beta-adrenergic agonist therapy. *Allergy Immunol Clin North Am* 1993;13:839-860.

12. Berenberg MJ, Baigelman W, Cupples LA, et al: Comparison of metered-dose inhaler attached to an Aerochamber with an updraft nebulizer for the administration of metaproterenol in hospitalized patients. *J Asthma* 1985;22:87-92.

13. Benton G, Thomas RC, Nickerson BG, et al: Experience with a metered-dose inhaler with a spacer in the pediatric emergency department. *Am J Dis Child* 1989;143:678-681.

14. Schuh S, Reisman J, Alshehri M, et al: A comparison of inhaled fluticasone and oral prednisone for children with severe acute asthma. *N Engl J Med* 2000;343:689-694.

15. Littenberg B, Gluck EH: A controlled trial of methylprednisolone in the emergency treatment of acute asthma. *N Engl J Med* 1986;314:150-152.

16. Qureshi F, et al: Effect of nebulized ipratropium on the hospitalization rates of children with asthma. *N Engl J Med* 1998; 339:1030-1035.

17. Littenberg B: Aminophylline treatment in severe, acute asthma. A meta-analysis. *JAMA* 1988;259:1678-1684.

18. Rodrigo C, Rodrigo G: Treatment of acute asthma. Lack of therapeutic benefit and increase the of toxicity from aminophylline given in addition to high doses of salbutamol deliverd by metered-dose inhaler with a spacer. *Chest* 1994;106:1071-1076.

19. Rowe BH, Bretzlaff JA, Bourdon C, et al: Intravenous magnesium sulfate treatment for acute asthma in the emergency department: a systematic review of the literature. *Ann Emerg Med* 2000;36:181-190.

20. Fitzgerald JM, Shragge D, Haddon J, et al: A randomized controlled trial of high-dose, inhaled budesonide versus oral prednisone in patients discharged form the emergency department following an acute asthma exacerbation. *Can Respir J* 2000;7:61-67.

21. Chapman KR, Verbeek PR, White JG, et al: Effect of a short course of prednisone in the prevention of early relapse after the emergency room treatment of acute asthma. *N Engl J Med* 1991; 324:788-794.

22. Enright PL, Lebowitz MD, Cockroft DW: Physiologic measures: pulmonary function tests. Asthma outcome. *Am J Respir Crit Care Med* 1994;149:S9-S18; discussion S19-S20.

23. Bryant DH, Rogers P: Effects of ipratropium bromide nebulizer solution with and without preservatives in the treatment of acute and stable asthma. *Chest* 1992;102:742-747.

24. Appel D, Karpel JP, Sherman M: Epinephrine improves expiratory flow rates in patients with asthma who do not respond to inhaled metaproterenol sulfate. *J Allergy Clin Immunol* 1989; 84:90-98.

25. National Asthma Education and Prevention Program, National Heart, Lung, and Blood Institute, National Institutes of Health: *Teach Your Patients About Asthma: A Clinician's Guide*. Bethesda, U.S. Department of Health and Human Services, 1992.

9

Urticaria and Angioedema

U rticaria (hives) and angioedema are common disorders, affecting about 25% of people sometime in their lives.[1] The intense itching and rapidly evolving lesions of urticaria can distress and frighten patients. Traditionally, urticaria that lasts less than 6 weeks is considered acute, while urticaria that lasts more than 6 weeks is designated chronic.[2] Many patients have intermittent episodes of acute urticaria separated by long periods of remission. Acute urticaria is commonly found in children and young adults, and reaches its peak prevalence in the third decade.[1] Chronic urticaria mainly affects middle-aged people, peaks in the fourth decade, and is more common in women than in men.

Mechanisms and Triggers of Urticaria and Angioedema

Urticaria and angioedema, which commonly coexist,[3] are caused by similar pathogenic mechanisms (Table 1). The main difference between these two disorders is in the location of the inflammation: urticaria primarily involves the dermis, while angioedema involves tissues under the skin.[4] Allergy is commonly implicated in acute urticaria, which can be triggered by foods, medications, or insect stings. A significant percentage of acute urticaria is caused by viral infections, especially in children.[4] In contrast to acute urticaria, no specific trigger is identified in 80% of patients with chronic urticaria.[3] Although the stimulus for chronic urticaria is unclear, the pathogenesis is related to infiltration of the skin by mast cells and mononuclear cells.[5,6] T cells constitute most of the mononuclear cell infiltrate and likely secrete histamine-releasing factors that promote mast cell mediator release. In acute allergic reactions, plasma histamine levels are elevated in 50% of cases and correlate with the extent of urticaria.[7] Autoimmune mechanisms have also been implicated in a subset of chronic urticaria patients who demonstrate autoantibodies that bind to the high-affinity immunoglobulin E (IgE) receptor.[2,8]

When a specific trigger for chronic urticaria is identified, physical stimuli are most often involved.[2,3,8] Dermatographism (acute pressure-induced urticaria), cholinergic urticaria (induced by passive heating, sweating, or fever), and cold-induced urticaria are the most common forms of physical urticaria.[3] Chronic urticaria can also be a manifestation of a systemic disease and occasionally is the presenting feature.[9,10] For example, chronic viral, parasitic, or bacterial infections are sometimes accompanied by generalized urticaria. Urticaria can also be the heralding sign of autoimmune disease such as systemic lupus erythematosus or thyroiditis. Finally, C1 esterase-inhibitor deficiency produces recurrent angioedema that is often triggered by minor trauma or surgery.[4,11]

Diagnosis

The most important factor in evaluating a patient with urticaria or angioedema is the medical history. Patients usually recognize food allergy when it triggers urticaria because the lesions typically appear within 30 minutes of ingesting the offending food, and this pattern occurs each time that food protein is ingested.[12,13] A similar temporal relationship usually exists when urticaria or angioedema is triggered by other allergic stimuli such as medications, la-

Table 1: Causes of Urticaria and Angioedema

Idiopathic

Allergic

- IgE-mediated
  - Foods, drugs, insect venoms, aeroallergens
- Anaphylactoid
  - Opiates, radiocontrast material
- Nonsteroidal anti-inflammatory drugs
- Serum-sickness reactions
- Contact urticaria

Physical stimuli

- Dermatographism
- Cholinergic urticaria
- Cold-induced urticaria
- Delayed pressure-induced urticaria
- Exercise
- Water
- Light
- Vibration

tex, or animals. In the case of serum sickness, however, hives and other signs and symptoms usually appear 7 to 14 days after a new medication or serum is started,[14] so the relationship is less obvious. Hives from occupational exposure typically flare while the patient is at work and then improve during weekends or vacations.[15]

The history is also the key factor in identifying physical urticaria, although specific tests are available to confirm the

Manifestation of systemic disease
- Infection
  - Viral, fungal, bacterial, parasitic
- Autoimmune
  - Urticaria vasculitis, systemic lupus erythematosus, thyroiditis, cryoglobulinemia
- Neoplasm
  - Lymphoma, leukemia
- Psychosomatic
- Mastocytosis

Toxic (acute urticaria or angioedema)
- Stinging nettles
- Fire coral

C1 esterase-inhibitor deficiency (angioedema)
- Hereditary
- Acquired

diagnosis (Table 2).[16,17] Dermatographism results from mast cells triggered by mild pressure, such as at the belt line or in intertrigo. Cholinergic urticaria often occurs when the core body temperature is raised by exercise, hot showers, or anxiety. A distinguishing factor in cholinergic urticaria is the appearance of the lesion, which is usually a punctate hive with surrounding erythema. Cold-induced urticaria typically occurs on body parts exposed to cold weather or after immer-

Table 2: Features of Common Types of Chronic Urticaria*

Type of urticaria	Age range (years)	Principal clinical features
Chronic idiopathic**	20-50	Profuse or sparse, generalized, pink, edematous papules or wheals, often annular, with itching
Symptomatic dermatographism	20-50	Itchy, linear wheals with surrounding bright red flare at sites of scratching or rubbing
Other physical urticarias		
Cold-induced	10-40	Itchy, pale, or red swelling at sites of contact with cold surfaces or fluids
Pressure-induced**	20-50	Large, painful, or itchy red swelling at sites of pressure (soles, palms, or waist) lasting 24 hours or more
Solar	20-50	Itchy, pale, or red swelling at site of exposure to ultraviolet or visible light
Cholinergic	10-50	Itching, monomorphic pale or pink wheals on trunk, neck, and limbs

* Modified from Greaves,[2] used with permission of the *New England Journal of Medicine* and the Massachusetts Medical Society, 1995;332:1767-1772.

Associated angioedema?	Diagnostic test
Yes	_____
No	Light stroking of skin causes an immediate wheal with itching.
Yes	Ten-minute application of an ice pack causes a wheal within 5 minutes of the removal of ice.
No	Application of pressure perpendicular to skin produces persistent red swelling after a latent period of 1-4 hours.
Yes	Irradiation by a 2.5-kW solar simulator (290-690 nm) for 30 to 120 seconds causes wheals within 30 minutes.
Yes	Exercise or a hot shower elicits an eruption.

** Pressure-induced and spontaneous wheals appear concurrently in 37% of patients with chronic idiopathic urticaria.

sion in cold water, which can sometimes produce massive urticaria and even anaphylaxis. Delayed pressure-induced urticaria and angioedema are more challenging to recognize because the onset of the swelling or skin lesions may occur several hours after strenuous physical exercise or application of pressure. The areas most commonly affected are the hands and feet, and pain is reported more often than itching. Less commonly, urticaria or angioedema can result from solar radiation, vibration, or contact with water.

On physical examination, the classic lesion of urticaria is a raised, pale area of dermal edema surrounded by a rim of erythema. In severe cases, the individual lesions coalesce into continuous skin lesions. As mentioned previously, the skin lesions of cholinergic urticaria have a distinct punctate appearance. Pruritus, present in most forms of urticaria, is important in distinguishing urticaria from skin disorders such as erythema multiforme that are similar in appearance.

Angioedema causes localized swelling and pallor of the involved subdermal tissues. The edematous tissues are soft and nonpitting and are not associated with lymphangitis. These features help to distinguish angioedema from other causes of dermal swelling such as infection or contact dermatitis. A diagnosis of C1 esterase-inhibitor deficiency should be considered in cases of recurrent angioedema, especially if there is also a history of recurrent abdominal pain, if angioedema is precipitated by trauma, or if the angioedema is not accompanied by urticarial lesions.

Another important clinical feature of urticaria and angioedema is that individual lesions tend to evolve and resolve quickly. Elias and colleagues[5] point out that hives caused by allergy tend to appear within minutes, while lesions of chronic urticaria evolve more slowly. In any case, individual urticarial lesions rarely last more than 24 hours and are not associated with any bruising or purpura; angioedema usually resolves within 24 to 72 hours. Individual urticarial lesions that persist for longer than 24 hours or are associated with purpura strongly suggest urticarial vasculitis,

Table 3: Laboratory Evaluation of Chronic Urticaria

- Complete blood count with differential
- Platelet count
- Sedimentation rate
- Antinuclear antibody
- Liver enzymes
- Urinalysis
- C4 level (for recurrent angioedema)
- Other tests as suggested by findings in the history and physical examination

and these circumstances should trigger a more extensive diagnostic evaluation, including biopsy of suspicious lesions.[18]

There are no characteristic laboratory features of urticaria or angioedema. Because an allergic cause is likely in acute urticaria or angioedema, allergen-specific skin tests or radioallergosorbent test (RAST) can be helpful in identifying causative factors. In contrast, skin tests are rarely useful in evaluating chronic urticaria. Because urticaria can be the presenting sign for a variety of systemic illnesses (Table 1), it is reasonable to order a limited panel of laboratory tests for patients with chronic urticaria or angioedema (Table 3). If there are indications of systemic illness, more extensive laboratory tests can help to determine the correct diagnosis.[9] If angioedema is recurrent, a C4 level should be obtained to screen for hereditary or acquired C1 esterase-inhibitor deficiency. This is addressed in greater detail later in this chapter.

Treatment of Urticaria and Angioedema

The treatment of acute and chronic urticaria and angioedema is outlined in Table 4. First, any factors that are

Table 4: Treatment of Chronic Urticaria

Avoid triggers
- Allergens, physical stimuli

Antihistamines
- H_1 blockers
- H_2 blockers

Corticosteroids (not for chronic therapy)
Other
- Doxepin
- Nifedipine (Adalat®, Procardia®)
- Cyclosporine (Sandimmune®)
- Intravenous immunoglobulin
- Ultraviolet A light +/- oral psoralen

known to cause the urticaria or angioedema must be avoided, including allergens, alcoholic beverages, and specific physical stimuli. Overly restricted diets should be discouraged unless there is clear evidence of food allergy.

The mainstay of medical therapy for angioedema and urticaria is the H_1-receptor antagonist.[19] For acute urticaria, it is best to use an antihistamine that has a rapid onset, such as diphenhydramine (Benadryl®) or hydroxyzine (Atarax®, Vistaril®), although sedation is a common side effect. For management of chronic urticaria (Figure 1), second-generation antihistamines are preferred because of their long half-lives and because they are either nonsedating (eg, loratadine [Claritin®]) or have a low incidence of sedation (eg, cetirizine [Zyrtec®]). In addition to H_1-antihistamines, tepid showers and the use of 1% menthol cream can provide symptomatic relief for acute outbreaks.

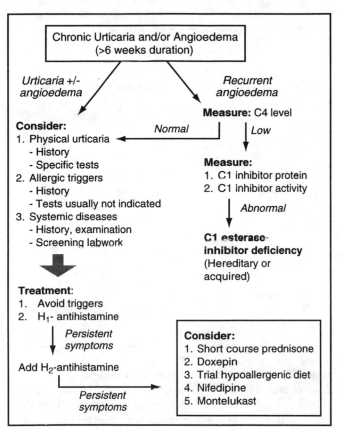

Figure 1: Management of chronic urticaria and angioedema.

Unfortunately, there are some patients with chronic urticaria who do not experience satisfactory relief with H_1-antihistamines alone. H_2-receptor blockers such as ranitidine (Zantac®) or cimetidine (Tagamet®) are often added to the medical regimen under these circumstances, but only 10% to 15% of patients experience additional relief.[20] Several other medications have been tried for patients with unremitting

Table 5: Complement Profiles With Angioedema*

Type	C1-Inh (antigenic)	C1-Inh (functional)	C1
HAE I	↓	↓	N
HAE II	N	↓	N
AAE I	↓	↓	↓
AAE II	N‡	↓	↓
Immune complex vasculitis	N	N	↓
Allergic/ idiopathic	N	N	N

‡Small decrease may be seen.

Abbreviations: N = normal, HAE = hereditary angioedema, AAE = acquired angioedema

urticaria. The addition of montelukast (Singulair®) can help control urticaria that is incompletely treated with antihistamines alone.[21] Doxepin (Sinequan®) is a tricyclic antidepressant that suppresses urticaria better than traditional antihistamines in some patients, but it frequently produces unpleasant side effects such as sedation and other central nervous system effects and drying of the mucous membranes. Nifedipine (Adalat®, Procardia®), a calcium-channel antagonist, significantly improved subjective and objective measures of chronic urticaria in one double-blind, placebo-controlled trial.[22] Cyclosporine, intravenous γ-globulin, and ultraviolet A (UVA) light with or without oral psoralen have all been used in a few patients with severe disease, with varying degrees of success.[23] For patients who have an au-

C4	C3	CH 50/100	Para-protein	Anti-C1-Inh Ab
↓	N	N‡	no	no
↓	N	N‡	no	no
↓	N‡	N‡	yes	no
↓	N‡	N‡	no	yes
↓	↓	↓	no	no
N	N	N	no	no

* Used with permission, from Huston DP, Bressler RB: *Med Clin North Am* 1992;76:805-840.

toantibody directed toward the high-affinity IgE receptor, plasmapheresis can induce clinical remission.[8,9] Oral glucocorticoids can be used to treat acute exacerbations of chronic urticaria, but they should not be used as maintenance medications because of the severe side effects that can be associated with long-term use.

C1 Esterase-Inhibitor Deficiency

C1 esterase-inhibitor deficiency can be inherited or acquired. Either form leads to unrestrained consumption of C2 and C4 and subsequent activation of the complement and plasma kinin-forming cascades.[4,10,11] Both disorders result in acute episodes of nonpruritic angioedema that are usually triggered by trauma, such as dental surgery. The resulting airway obstruction can be life threatening. In addition, edema of the intestines produces episodes of vomiting, severe abdominal pain, and intestinal obstruction. Urticarial lesions are generally not found in patients with hereditary or acquired C1 esterase-inhibitor deficiency.

Hereditary angioedema is transmitted as an autosomal dominant trait, and two forms have been identified: type 1, where there is an absolute deficiency of the C1 esterase-inhibitor protein; and type 2, where the C1 esterase inhibitor is present but nonfunctional. Acquired C1 inhibitor deficiency is most often associated with B-cell lymphoproliferative disorders. A second form has been described in which serum autoantibodies to C1 inhibitor interfere with its functional activity.

Screening for C1 esterase deficiency is accomplished by performing quantitative measurements of C4, which is decreased even in the absence of angioedema (Table 5). It is important to realize that C1 esterase-inhibitor deficiency is associated with angioedema but not urticaria and that C4 levels are normal in patients who present with both angioedema and urticaria. The two forms of hereditary angioedema can be distinguished by assaying for C1 esterase-inhibitor protein levels and C1 esterase-inhibitor activity. Patients with acquired C1 esterase-inhibitor deficiency should be evaluated for a B-cell lymphoproliferative disorder, and serum should be screened for autoantibodies specific for C1 esterase inhibitor.

Treatment of C1 esterase-inhibitor deficiency consists of three separate strategies: long-term prophylaxis, short-term prophylaxis, and treatment of acute attacks.[4,10,11] Because the degree of C1 esterase-inhibitor activity varies in affected patients, long-term prophylaxis is not required for all patients. The drugs that are most helpful for prophylaxis are androgens such as danazol (Danocrine®) or stanozolol (Winstrol®), which stimulate C1 esterase-inhibitor synthesis in the liver. Antifibrinolytic drugs such as ε-aminocaproic acid (Amicar®) and tranexamic acid (Cyklokapron®) have also been used for long-term prophylaxis, but their use is limited by side effects such as thrombosis and myonecrosis.

Short-term prophylaxis is used to prepare a patient for traumatic procedures such as dental surgery. Purified C1 esterase inhibitor is the most effective treatment agent for short-term prophylaxis or for acute attacks of angioedema, but, if this is not available, fresh frozen plasma can also be used. Some patients with acquired C1 esterase-inhibitor deficiency develop a partial resistance to C1 inhibitor infusion but usually respond to larger doses.

References

1. Schafer T, Ring J: Epidemiology of urticaria. *Monogr Allergy* 1993;31:49-60.

2. Greaves MW: Chronic urticaria. *N Engl J Med* 1995;332: 1767 1772.

3. Champion RH, Roberts SO, Carpenter RG, et al: Urticaria and angio-oedema. A review of 554 patients. *Br J Dermatol* 1969; 81:588-597.

4. Huston DP, Bressler RB: Urticaria and angioedema. *Med Clin North Am* 1992;76:805-840.

5. Elias J, Boss E, Kaplan AP: Studies of the cellular infiltrate of chronic idiopathic urticaria: prominence of T-lymphocytes, monocytes, and mast cells. *J Allergy Clin Immunol* 1986;78: 914-918.

6. Barlow RJ, Ross EL, MacDonald DM, et al: Mast cells and T lymphocytes in chronic urticaria. *Clin Exp Allergy* 1995;25:317-322.

7. Lin RY, Schwartz LB, Curry A, et al: Histamine and tryptase levels in patients with acute allergic reactions: an emergency department-based study. *J Allergy Clin Immunol* 2000;106:65-71.

8. Hide M, Francis DM, Grattan CE, et al: Autoantibodies against the high-affinity IgE receptor as a cause of histamine release in chronic urticaria. *N Engl J Med* 1993;328:1599-1604.

9. Greaves M: Chronic urticaria. *J Allergy Clin Immunol* 2000; 105:664-672.

10. Stafford CT: Urticaria as a sign of systemic disease. *Ann Allergy* 1990;64:264-270.

11. Carreer FM: The C1 inhibitor deficiency. A review. *Eur J Clin Chem Clin Biochem* 1992;30:793-807.

12. Bock SA, Atkins FM: Patterns of food hypersensitivity during sixteen years of double-blind, placebo-controlled oral food challenges. *J Pediatr* 1990;117:561-567.

13. Sampson HA, McCaskill CM: Food hypersensitivity and atopic dermatitis: evaluation of 113 patients. *J Pediatr* 1985;107: 669-675.

14. Lawley TJ, Bielory L, Gascon P, et al: A prospective clinical and immunologic analysis of patients with serum sickness. *N Engl J Med* 1984;311:1407-1413.

15. Mathias CG: Occupational dermatoses. *J Am Acad Dermatol* 1988;19:1107-1114.

16. Mahmood T: Physical urticarias. *Am Fam Physician* 1994; 49:1411-1414.

17. Greaves MW: The physical urticarias. *Clin Exp Allergy* 1991; 21:284-289.

18. Mortureux P, Leaute-Labreze C, Legrain-Lifermann V, et al: Acute urticaria in infancy and early childhood: a prospective study. *Arch Dermatol* 1998;134:319-323.

19. Simons FE, Simons KJ: The pharmacology and use of H_1-receptor-antagonist drugs. *N Engl J Med* 1994;330:1663-1670.

20. Paul E, Bodeker RH: Treatment of chronic urticaria with terfenadine and ranitidine. A randomized double-blind study in 45 patients. *Eur J Clin Pharmacol* 1986;31:277-280.

21. Erbagei Z: The leukotriene receptor antagonist montelukast in the treatment of chronic idiopathic urticaria: a single-blind, placebo-controlled crossover clinical study. *J Allergy Clin Immunol* 2002;110:484-488.

22. Bressler RB, Sowell K, Huston DP: Therapy of chronic idiopathic urticaria with nifedipine: demonstration of beneficial effect in a double-blind, placebo-controlled, crossover trial. *J Allergy Clin Immunol* 1989;83:756-763.

23. Kennard CD, Ellis CN: Pharmacologic therapy for urticaria. *J Am Acad Dermatol* 1991;25:176-189.

10

Atopic and Contact Dermatitis

A topic dermatitis and contact dermatitis are common allergic inflammatory disorders of the superficial layer of the skin and are associated with intense pruritus. Despite these similarities, the pathologic mechanisms, natural history, distribution of lesions, and treatments for each disorder are quite different. This chapter reviews the clinical features and therapy for each of these disorders.

Atopic Dermatitis

Atopic dermatitis is a chronic skin disorder characterized by pruritus, dry skin, and excoriation, which may be localized to a few patches or involve large portions of the body. Atopic dermatitis tends to occur in individuals who have a personal or family history of allergic rhinitis, asthma, or eczema,[1] and it is most common in children. As with the other atopic diseases, its incidence appears to be increasing, and recent studies have estimated that between 10% and 20% of children are affected in most Western countries.[2,3]

Early lesions of atopic dermatitis are red and dry with small papules, mild scaling, and areas of excoriation. Chronically affected areas show accentuated skin lines and thickening of the skin (lichenification). Postinflammatory pigmentation abnormalities are common. Pruritus is universally present, and scratching is a major factor in the pathogenesis of acute and chronic skin lesions. Moist and oozing lesions are also common and suggest the possibility of superficial infection.

Several features of the natural history of atopic dermatitis are distinctive. Atopic dermatitis usually begins early in life, typically in the second 6 months of the first year. The pattern of distribution of atopic dermatitis lesions changes with age. Affected areas in infants include the cheeks, trunk, and extensor surfaces of the extremities. During childhood and adolescence, the distribution shifts to the flexural areas of the extremities and neck. The hands and feet may also be involved and, in fact, this may be the only manifestation of atopic dermatitis in some patients. In addition, there appears to be seasonal variation in severity, which tends to worsen in the dry winter months. As with other atopic diseases, the severity of atopic dermatitis tends to decrease after childhood, although increased skin sensitivity and occasional outbreaks of localized disease persist in most patients. However, active disease can be extremely uncomfortable and unsightly, and this underscores the importance of education and preventive therapy for this chronic disease.

A complication associated with atopic dermatitis is an increased susceptibility to skin infections, especially those involving *Staphylococcus* or *Streptococcus*. Herpes simplex infection may also be troublesome in patients with atopic dermatitis, and topical or oral treatment with acyclovir (Zovirax®) may be necessary for persistent or severe lesions. Severe atopic dermatitis may also be complicated by psychologic problems,[4] decreased growth velocity,[5] and cataracts.[6]

The pathogenesis of atopic dermatitis has not been clearly defined. The wide range in prevalence of ectopic dermatitis among countries inhabited by similar ethnic groups suggests that environmental factors play a major role in determining the risk of the disorder.[3] Histologic features include intracellular edema (spongiosis) with formation of vesicles, hyperplasia of the epidermis, infiltration of inflammatory cells such as lymphocytes and macrophages in acute lesions, and epidermal thickening and fibrosis in chronic lesions.[2] Circulating eosinophil counts are commonly elevated and correlate with disease severity.[7] Finally, certain bacterial proteins such as staphylococcal and streptococcal toxins may contribute to the pathogenesis of atopic dermatitis through superantigen activation of T cells in the skin,[8] and there is evidence that atopic dermatitis is associated with reduced levels of endogenous antibacterial peptides in the skin.[9]

Diagnosis

Atopic dermatitis is a clinical diagnosis based on the typical appearance and clinical course of the disorder. Distinguishing features of atopic dermatitis include the early age of onset; the distribution of the lesions, with characteristic shifting in distribution between infancy and later childhood; coexistence with other atopic diseases; the chronic nature of the disorder; and the prominent symptom of pruritus. Although circulating eosinophil counts and serum immunoglobulin E (IgE) levels are commonly elevated in atopic dermatitis, these findings are not specific and are usually not helpful in establishing the diagnosis.

Identifying factors that trigger flares of atopic dermatitis (Table 1) is essential in designing a rational treatment regimen. Sudden worsening of atopic dermatitis strongly suggests superficial bacterial infection of the skin. This is usually accompanied by a dramatic increase in pruritus, and the lesions may appear red, crusted, or weepy.

Irritants, including detergents, perfume, or other skin care products, can also trigger acute symptoms. It is important to consider handwashing habits because frequent abrasion from washing and drying the skin can produce local outbreaks of eczema. Occupational exposure to food prod-

Table 1: Triggers of Atopic Dermatitis

Abrasion
- Scratching
- Rough clothing

Infection
- *Staphylococcus*
- *Streptococcus*

Allergens
- Food (in children)
- Epidermal allergens
  - House dust mite

Climate
- Cold, dry winter air

Stress

Sweating

Contact dermatitis

ucts, plant material, and the handling of other proteins or chemicals can cause atopic dermatitis, contact urticaria, or contact dermatitis. Allergic contact dermatitis, which is addressed in the second half of this chapter, can also trigger pruritus and eczema.

Studies have shown that food allergy is key in the pathogenesis of atopic dermatitis in some infants and young children and that it is especially common in children with severe disease that is relatively unresponsive to traditional therapy.[10] Allergic reactions to food often involve several organ systems, most commonly the skin, the gastrointestinal tract, and the respiratory system. Skin manifestations, such as flushing, urticaria, and angioedema, tend to occur soon after the offending food is eaten. In contrast, changes in atopic dermatitis typically appear hours or days after food ingestion, which makes it more difficult to identify the offending allergen. Evaluation involves a careful history and testing for food-specific IgE by either radioallergosorbent test (RAST) or skin testing. False-positive skin test or RAST results are common. Blinded food challenges can be helpful in determining the validity of these test results.[11] Food allergy associated with eczema seems to be uncommon in adults.

Several investigators have suggested that respiratory allergens, such as house dust mite or pollens, may contribute to the pathogenesis of atopic dermatitis,[12,13] and measures directed at decreasing the levels of house dust mite allergen in the environment have produced dramatic clinical improvement in some cases. Patch testing using epidermal allergens can be performed, but the clinical relevance of these tests has not been clearly defined.[14] It remains to be determined if this association is limited to a small number of patients or is a more common phenomenon.

Treatment

Treatment of atopic dermatitis involves maintaining good skin hygiene, avoiding factors known to trigger symptoms, and treating flares of dermatitis when they occur. As is the case with most chronic diseases, patient education must be stressed to achieve optimum results. General measures that may be helpful in the long-term control of atopic dermatitis include the use of skin moisturizers and avoiding heavy or irritating fabric, such as woolen clothes, because these may trigger scratching and, thus, skin rash. Frequent bathing followed by the immediate (within 2 to 3 minutes) application of moisturizing creams or ointments moisturizes the skin and reduces the risk of secondary bacterial infections.

Topical corticosteroids are used to maintain healthy skin and to treat exacerbations of dermatitis.[2,15] A low-potency corticosteroid (Table 2) such as 1% hydrocortisone cream (Hytone®) can be applied to affected areas of the skin twice daily for mild manifestations of atopic dermatitis. Medium-potency corticosteroids, such as 0.025% to 0.1% triamcinolone (Aristocort®, Kenalog®) can be used to treat localized patches of more severely affected skin. Facial skin is highly vascular, leading to great absorption of topical corticoster-

Table 2: Classification of Selected Topical Corticosteroids by Potency

Class	Corticosteroid	Brand names
I (strongest)	betamethasone dipropionate 0.05%	Diprolene®
	clobetasol propionate 0.05%	Temovate®
	halobetasol propionate 0.05%	Ultravate®
II	fluocinonide 0.05%	Lidex®
	desoximetasone 0.25%	Topicort®
III	triamcinolone acetonide 0.1%	Aristocort®, Kenalog®
	mometasone furoate 0.1%	Elocon®
	fluocinolone acetonide 0.025%	Synalar®
IV	triamcinolone acetonide 0.025%	Aristocort®, Kenalog®
	hydrocortisone valerate 0.2%	Westcort®
	hydrocortisone butyrate 0.1%	Locoid®
V	alclometasone dipropionate 0.05%	Aclovate®
	desonide 0.05%	DesOwen®
	fluocinolone acetonide 0.01%	Tridesilon® Synalar®
VI (weakest)	hydrocortisone 1%, 2.5%	Hytone®

oids and increased susceptibility to side effects such as skin atrophy, striae, or telangiectasia. Therefore, corticosteroid use on the face should be restricted to low-potency preparations such as 1% hydrocortisone (Table 2). Intertriginous areas such as the groin and axilla are also more sensitive to corticosteroid side effects.

Corticosteroid skin preparations are classified by potency (Table 2), and clinicians should become familiar with one or two in each of the classes. High-potency (class I or II) corticosteroids are rarely needed in the treatment of atopic dermatitis. Patients who initially respond to one particular cream may develop tolerance to it and can benefit from the use of a different corticosteroid of the same potency. Contact dermatitis caused by hypersensitivity to a topical corticosteroid is another cause of treatment failure.[16]

For patients with severe atopic dermatitis that is refractory to standard therapy, the use of 0.03% to 0.1% tacrolimus (FK506) ointment (Protopic®) or pimecrolimus 1% cream (Elidel®) can produce marked improvement in skin signs and symptoms.[17] Fortunately, these medications do not inhibit collagen synthesis, so their use is not associated with atrophic skin changes. Side effects can include burning of the skin after application, which is more common with tacrolimus, and increased severity of cutaneous viral infections (eg, herpes simplex).

In addition to moisturization and corticosteroid creams, oral antihistamines can be helpful in controlling pruritus. Hydroxyzine (Atarax®, Vistaril®) is particularly effective in controlling pruritus, but sedation often limits clinical usefulness. One approach to lessen this side effect is to give hydroxyzine as a single nighttime dose[18] (50 mg in adults or 1 to 2 mg/kg in children). If standard antihistamines are ineffective or if they produce drowsiness, a nonsedating antihistamine such as loratadine (Claritin®) should be prescribed. Use of topical antihistamines (eg, lotions containing diphenhydramine) should be avoided because of the high incidence of contact dermatitis associated with these preparations.

Acute Exacerbations of Atopic Dermatitis

Acute flares of atopic dermatitis should be treated with a combination of anti-infective therapy and intense local skin care (Table 3). Localized breakouts of atopic dermatitis should be cleaned and hydrated either by bathing or by wrapping a wet towel around the affected area for 15 or 20 minutes 2 to 3 times a day, followed immediately by the application of a moisturizing cream or ointment and a medium-potency corticosteroid. Infection should be strongly suspected in cases characterized by a sudden dramatic increase in severity, especially if the skin lesions are very red, weepy, or crusted. Surface cultures of the skin should be obtained because of the increasing frequency of antibiotic-resistant bacteria. Institution of antibiotic therapy (eg, erythromycin, cephalexin [Keflex®]) directed at *Staphylococcus* and *Streptococcus* often produces dramatic resolution of the skin rash within 2 to 3 days.

Systemic corticosteroids can be considered in some cases of acute severe outbreaks of eczema. However, their use should be avoided in the daily management of this disorder because of the significant side affects associated with long-term corticosteroid use.

Contact Dermatitis

Contact dermatitis is a common skin disease caused by exposure to irritants or allergens, producing skin inflammation and pruritus that is usually limited to the area of exposure.[19] The lesions are characterized by erythema, superficial edema that produces a firm texture, and vesiculation that typically begins with microvesicles that may coalesce to form larger blisters. Unroofing of the vesicles through scratching results in weeping and crusting of the lesions. Although the clinical appearance of the individual lesions is nonspecific, the distribution of skin lesions is usually diagnostic because it corresponds with the application of the inciting agent.

Different mechanisms are responsible for allergic and irritant contact dermatitis.[19,20] Allergic contact dermatitis

Table 3: Management of Acute Flares of Atopic Dermatitis

- Administer soaking baths* in cool or lukewarm water for 20 minutes twice daily, then:

- Immediately apply medium-potency topical corticosteroid (eg, 0.025%-0.1% triamcinolone cream) to affected skin, except the face, and

- Immediately apply 1% hydrocortisone cream to facial rash or less severely affected areas of the skin, and

- Immediately apply a moisturizing cream or ointment to other areas of dry skin.

- Prescribe antistaphylococcal antibiotic therapy for severe flares, or for those accompanied by lesions that are weeping or crusted or have marked erythema.

    Consider performing skin culture when prescribing antistaphylococcal therapy because of the prevalence of resistant bacterial strains.

- Prescribe an antihistamine (eg, hydroxyzine, a nonsedating antihistamine) for relief of pruritus.

- Schedule a follow-up visit to assess improvement and adjust the maintenance regimen as needed.

* For localized eruptions, as a substitute for bathing, the affected area may be wrapped in a wet cloth for 20 minutes.

is caused by a type IV hypersensitivity reaction involving sensitization of allergen-specific T cells in regional lymph nodes. The sensitized T cells home back to the skin and are reactivated by the contact allergen to secrete cytokines that activate macrophages and other effector cells at the site of inflammation.[21] The activated cells in the skin cause the dermatitis. In contrast, irritant dermatitis does not involve an immunologic mechanism and instead results from contact with a substance that damages, or irritates, the skin. Consequently, an irritant can cause dermatitis after the first exposure because no period of sensitization is required.

Because immunologic sensitization is a prerequisite to the development of allergic contact dermatitis, it follows that the rate of sensitization largely depends on the frequency and duration of exposure to potential allergens. For example, Europeans are not sensitive to poison ivy or poison oak because these are 'New World' plants. As another example, the rate of nickel sensitivity is up to 10 times higher in women, presumably because of increased exposure to nickel-containing alloys in jewelry.[22]

Treatment of allergic contact dermatitis is based on avoidance of the inciting agent, so it is essential to carefully evaluate the history and pattern of distribution of skin lesions to identify the allergen. Clinicians should 'step into the patient's shoes' to obtain a complete history of daily activities, including the use of cosmetics, toiletries, hair preparations and dyes, and topical medications. Occupational exposures are important, as many industrial chemicals, proteins, and irritants have been implicated in contact dermatitis.[19,23] In fact, skin-related complaints account for up to 90% of all claims for workers' compensation.[23] Exposure to potential allergens through hobbies and housework should also be explored. Finally, because many topical medications cause contact dermatitis, it is crucial to get a complete history of the treatments that have been used on the rash.

Common skin sensitizers and their sources are listed in Table 4.[19,22,24] The association of a known skin sensitizer with the onset of a localized dermatitis establishes a provisional diagnosis, and presumptive therapy can then be started. However, contact dermatitis often follows the application of preparations with many ingredients, making it difficult to identify the offending allergen. In this situation,

Table 4: Causes of Contact Dermatitis

A. Irritant dermatitis

- Soaps, detergents
- Abrasion (handwashing)
- Occlusion
- Acids
- Alkali
- Solvents

B. Allergic contact dermatitis

Source	Allergen
Topical medicines	Neomycin
	Bacitracin
	Benzocaine
	Corticosteroids
	Diphenhydramine
Medicine or cosmetic additives	Thimerosal
	Quaternium-15
	Fragrances
	Balsam of Peru
	Formaldehyde
	Lanolin
Sunscreen	PABA
Jewelry	Nickel
Pocket change	Cobalt
Belt buckles	
Hair dye	Paraphenylenediamine
Cement, leather	Dichromate
Plants	Various
Shoes	Thiuram
Rubber products	Stabilizers

patch testing can be used to identify the allergen, opening the way to effective treatment and avoidance measures. Despite recent advances in the standardization of allergen preparations and techniques,[19,24] patch testing is still very much an art and should only be performed by physicians formally trained in this technique. There are many causes of false-positive and false-negative results,[25] and these limitations are even more evident when testing with materials that have not been standardized. Regrettably, this is often necessary because of the limited number of commercially available standardized extracts.

Treatment

The primary treatment for allergic contact dermatitis is avoidance of the allergen, but lesions may persist for weeks without additional anti-inflammatory therapy. Corticosteroids speed the resolution of skin lesions and associated symptoms. If topical therapy is used, we advise prescribing a class I or class II corticosteroid (Table 2), but therapy should be limited to 2 weeks to avoid cutaneous side effects. In addition, potent corticosteroid preparations should never be used on the face because of the high incidence of side effects. For severe outbreaks of contact dermatitis on the body, or moderate to severe lesions on the face, oral corticosteroids are the most effective treatment,[26] if there are no medical contraindications. A 2- to 3-week course of prednisone, starting with 40 to 60 mg/d in adults or 1 mg/kg/d in children given in split doses followed by a slow taper, produces satisfactory relief in most patients. However, relapses are common if the prednisone is tapered over a shorter time.

Other supportive measures include the use of cool compresses with either Burow's solution or saline to relieve local discomfort, cleaning the affected area, and speed-drying of the lesions. Antihistamines such as hydroxyzine can be used to treat pruritus, although topical antihistamine or anesthetic agents should be avoided because they are potent skin sensitizers. Secondary bacterial infections should be treated with oral antibiotics with good coverage of staphylococcal and streptococcal bacteria.

References

1. Dold S, Wjst M, von Mutius E, et al: Genetic risk for asthma, allergic rhinitis, and atopic dermatitis. *Arch Dis Child* 1992; 67:1018-1022.

2. Schultz Larsen F: Atopic dermatitis: an increasing problem. *Pediatr Allergy Immunol* 1996;7:51-53.

3. Williams H, Robertson C, Stewart A, et al: Worldwide variations in the prevalence of symptoms of atopic eczema in the international study of asthma and allergies in childhood. *J Allergy Clin Immunol* 1999:103:125-138.

4. Daud LR, Garralda ME, David TJ: Psychosocial adjustment in preschool children with atopic eczema. *Arch Dis Child* 1993; 69:670-676.

5. Massarano AA, Hollis S, Devlin J, et al: Growth in atopic eczema. *Arch Dis Child* 1993;68:677-679.

6. Niwa Y, Iizawa O: Abnormalities in serum lipids and leukocyte superoxide dismutase and associated cataract formation in patients with atopic dermatitis. *Arch Dermatol* 1994;130: 1387-1392.

7. Magnarin M, Knowles A, Ventura A, et al: A role for eosinophils in the pathogenesis of skin lesions in patients with food-sensitive atopic dermatitis. *J Allergy Clin Immunol* 1995;96: 200-208.

8. Leung DY: Atopic dermatitis: new insights and opportunities for therapist intervention. *J Allergy Clin Immunol* 2000;105:860-870.

9. Ong PY, Ohtake T, Brandt C, et al: Endogenous antimicrobial peptides and skin infections in atopic dermatitis. *N Engl J Med* 2002;347:1151-1160.

10. Sampson HA, McCaskill CC: Food hypersensitivity and atopic dermatitis: evaluation of 113 patients. *J Pediatr* 1985;107: 669-675.

11. Bock SA, Sampson HA, Atkins FM, et al: Double-blind, placebo-controlled food challenge (DBPCFC) as an office procedure: a manual. *J Allergy Clin Immunol* 1988;82:986-987.

12. Norris PG, Schofield O, Camp RD: A study of the role of house dust mite in atopic dermatitis. *Br J Dermatol* 1988;118: 435-440.

13. Adinoff AD, Tellez P, Clark RA: Atopic dermatitis and aeroallergen contact sensitivity. *J Allergy Clin Immunol* 1988;81: 736-742.

14. Darsow U, Vieluf D, Ring J: Atopy patch test with different vehicles and allergen concentrations: an approach to standardization. *J Allergy Clin Immunol* 1995;95:677-684.

15. McHenry PM, Williams HC, Bingham EA: Management of atopic eczema. Joint Workshop of the British Association of Dermatologists and the Research Unit of the Royal College of Physicians of London. *BMJ* 1995;310:843-847.

16. Rietschel RL: Patch testing for corticosteroid allergy in the United States. *Arch Dermatol* 1995;131:91-92.

17. Bieber T: Topical tacrolimus (FK506): a new milestone in the management of atopic dermatitis. *J Allergy Clin Immunol* 1998; 102:555-557.

18. Goetz DW, Jacobson JM, Apaliski SJ, et al: Objective antihistamine side effects are mitigated by evening dosing of hydroxyzine. *Ann Allergy* 1991;67:448-454.

19. Rietschel RL: Occupational contact dermatitis. *Lancet* 1997; 349:1093-1095.

20. Traidl C, Sebastiani S, Albanesi C, et al: Disparate cytotoxic activity of nickel-specific CD8+ and CD4+ T cell subsets against keratinocytes. *J Immunol* 2000;165:3058-3064.

21. Zanni MP, Mauri-Hellweg D, Brander C, et al: Characterization of lidocaine-specific T cells. *J Immunol* 1997;158: 1139-1148.

22. Marks JG, Belsito DV, DeLeo VA, et al: North American Contact Dermatitis Group: patch test results for the detection of delayed-type hypersensitivity to topical allergens. *J Am Acad Dermatol* 1998;38:911-918.

23. Mathias CG: Occupational dermatoses. *J Am Acad Dermatol* 1988;19:1107-1114.

24. Brasch J, Henseler T, Aberer W, et al: Reproducibility of patch tests. A multicenter study of synchronous left- versus right-sided patch tests by the German Contact Dermatitis Research Group. *J Am Acad Dermatol* 1994;31:584-591.

25. Oshima H, Kawahara D, Hashimoto Y, et al: An approach to evaluating patch test results. *Contact Dermatitis* 1994;31: 189-191.

26. Spector SL: Oral steroid therapy for asthma and contact dermatitis. *JAMA* 1992;268:1926.

11

Food Allergy

O f all the forms of allergy, perhaps none is more misunderstood by the general public than food allergy. This is undoubtedly because of the large volume of misinformation about food allergy that has been published in the popular press, as well as a history of confusing and conflicting reports published in the medical literature. Recent advances in the identification, purification, and standardization of food allergens, as well as improved diagnostic techniques, such as the double-blind, placebo-controlled food challenge, have provided new insights about the nature of food allergy. Consequently, these insights have led to the development of rational approaches to the diagnosis of food allergy.

It is important to understand the difference between the two types of adverse reaction to foods—food *allergy* and food *intolerance*. Food allergy is caused by an immunologic reaction to a specific food protein. In most cases, this involves an immunoglobulin E (IgE)-mediated type I hypersensitivity reaction, although less common forms of food allergy do not involve IgE.[1-3] In contrast, food intolerance may stem from one of a number of different nonimmunologic mechanisms (Table 1). Examples of food intolerance include lactose intolerance, resulting in an inability to digest the ma-

Table 1: Food Intolerances

Metabolic deficiencies
- Lactase deficiency
- Phenylketonuria

Pharmacologic properties of food
- Caffeine → insomnia
- Serotonin → migraine headaches

Food poisoning
- Histamine (scombroid fish)
- Staphylococcal enterotoxin

Irritant reactions
- Capsaicin → heartburn
- Sulfites → bronchospasm

jor sugar in milk; food poisoning, which may be caused by toxins or microbes contaminating the food; or pharmacologic reactions to food ingredients, such as sleeplessness caused by the ingestion of caffeine. Scombroid fish poisoning is an example of a food poisoning that closely mimics an allergic reaction. In this case, the breakdown of histidine contained in the dark meat of deep-swimming ocean fish such as tuna or swordfish causes a buildup of histamine within the fish.[4] Ingestion of fish containing large amounts of histamine can produce symptoms that are almost indistinguishable from those caused by allergy, including gastrointestinal distress, flushing, urticaria, respiratory distress, and even hypotension.

Several important distinctions exist between food intolerance and food allergy. First, food allergic reactions are precipitated by food proteins, of which only a very small amount is needed to set off an allergic reaction. In contrast, people with food intolerance are often able to ingest a small

Table 2: Clinical Manifestations of Food Allergy

Allergic syndrome	Organ system
IgE-mediated	Skin
	Gastrointestinal
	Respiratory
	Neurologic
	Cardiovascular
Non-IgE immune mechanism	Gastrointestinal
	Cardiovascular

amount of the offending food and develop symptoms only if larger amounts are eaten. For instance, most people with lactose intolerance can drink up to several ounces of milk without experiencing any adverse reactions. Furthermore, allergic reactions are reproducible because they occur after eating or drinking any food containing the offending food protein. For instance, a person allergic to milk protein will

Rapid onset	Delayed onset
Urticaria	Eczema
Angioedema	
Flushing	
Pruritus	
Mouth pruritus	Failure to thrive
Vomiting	Iron deficiency
Abdominal pain	Protcin loss
Diarrhea	
Rhinorrhea	↑ Asthma
Tearing	
Wheezing	
Laryngeal edema	
Migraine (rare)	
Seizures (rare)	
Shock	Shock
Hematochezia	Iron deficiency
Vomiting	Protein loss
Abdominal pain	Failure to thrive
Diarrhea	
Hypovolemia	Hypovolemia
Shock	

experience symptoms after drinking milk or eating ice cream, cheese, or butter. In contrast, a person with lactose intolerance may be able to tolerate yogurt, which contains less lactose than milk, whereas drinking a similar amount of whole milk may lead to gastrointestinal symptoms.

Surveys have revealed that approximately 30% of people believe that they or their children are allergic to one or more foods, but the true incidence of food allergy is much lower.[5] Studies using double-blind, placebo-controlled food challenges indicate that between 2% and 7.5% of children actually have food allergy, and the incidence in adults is believed to be significantly lower.[6] Presumably, the remainder of these self-reported reactions are caused by food intolerance or are mistakenly identified as food-caused symptoms. Overdiagnosis of food allergy is undesirable because it can lead to needless dietary restriction and, in some cases, to nutritional deficiencies.[7]

Clinical Manifestations

Historical information, such as the timing of symptoms in relation to food ingestion and the organ systems affected, provides important clues about whether an adverse reaction is from food allergy, food intolerance, or some other cause. Allergic reactions typically occur soon after the ingestion of the offending food, often within minutes and nearly always within 2 hours.[8,9] Delayed reactions, although uncommon, can occur if food absorption is delayed or if the allergic reaction is from a mechanism other than type I hypersensitivity.[1,3]

Food allergy can affect several different organ systems, including the gastrointestinal tract, the skin, the cardiovascular system, the respiratory tract, and the central nervous system (Table 2).[3,6,8,10] The gastrointestinal tract and the skin are the most commonly affected organ systems. Many people with food allergy develop unpleasant sensations in the mouth, such as itching, burning, or tingling, within seconds after ingesting the food. Abdominal pain, nausea, vomiting, and diarrhea are common gastrointestinal symptoms. Cutaneous manifestations of food allergy include urticaria, angioedema, and flushing, especially of the face, neck, and ears. Patients with atopic dermatitis may experience a generalized itching sensation after ingesting a food allergen. This may be followed hours later by an increase in the severity of eczema.[9] Respiratory symptoms are the next most common manifestation of food allergy. These may range from mild symptoms, such as watering of the eyes and rhinorrhea, to severe bronchospasm or obstruction of the upper airway. Upper airway obstruction may be insidious in nature and may begin with mild symptoms such as hoarseness of the voice or slight swelling of the tongue. These symptoms may progress either rapidly or over several hours to produce severe respiratory distress. It is unusual, however, for respiratory symptoms to be the only manifestation of food allergy.[11]

Life-threatening allergic reactions to food may also involve the cardiovascular system, producing capillary leakage, diminished cardiac output, and hypotension. Three different patterns can be observed with an allergic reaction to food.[12,13] The first pattern is typical of an immediate response, with symptoms appearing within minutes of food ingestion and resolving within 30 minutes to 1 hour. Biphasic responses may also be observed, in which symptoms are initially prominent, followed in succession by a quiescent period and then reappearance of symptoms. Finally, some reactions begin with mild manifestations that progressively worsen over several hours. Thus, it is important not to underestimate the severity of a reaction simply because the initial manifestations are mild.

The potential association between food allergy and neurologic reactions precipitated by food allergy has generated considerable controversy. Migraine headaches can be triggered by the ingestion of foods such as chocolate and aged cheeses, although this association is probably due to a pharmacologic rather than an allergic response to the food. There are also a few case reports of seizures caused by food allergy. The use of diets restricted in sugar and food additives (eg, the Finegold diet), or oligoallergenic diets in the treatment of attention deficit disorder or other behavioral disorders have not been validated and should be avoided.[14-16] Multiple vague complaints, such as lethargy and headache, in the absence of signs or symptoms of hypersensitivity are unlikely to be caused by food allergy.[17]

Food-induced enterocolitis syndrome is an example of a food allergy that occurs independently of food-specific IgE, as skin and radioallergosorbent tests (RAST) are usually negative.[1,18] This disorder occurs most often in 3- to 6-month-old infants, and symptoms develop 4 to 6 hours after ingestion of formulas containing either soy or milk protein. Affected infants develop gastrointestinal symptoms, including vomiting, hematochezia, diarrhea, and hypovolemia. Chronic allergen exposure may produce anemia, failure to thrive, and hypovolemia. Celiac disease is another non-IgE-mediated disorder in which an immunologic reaction to grain glutens produces mucosal damage to the small intestine that leads to chronic malabsorption.[3]

Diagnosing Food Allergy

Systematic evaluation of data obtained with the history and physical examination, along with determination of food-specific IgE and food challenge procedures, can be used to accurately diagnose food allergy (Table 3).[6,19] Historical information should be evaluated with a few key points in mind, including the timing of the adverse reaction in relation to when the food was ingested; the reproducibility of the adverse reaction after repeat exposure to the same food protein; and the involvement of the typical organ systems as described previously. Physical examination is important to exclude other possibilities in the differential diagnosis, such as primary gastrointestinal disorders. Testing for food-specific IgE using either prick skin testing or RAST can provide valuable data to support or disprove the possibility of food allergy. However, it is important to realize the limitations of these tests. Both tests have a high (>90% for most allergens) negative predictive value and can reliably exclude the possibility of IgE-mediated food allergy,[20] although it is important to remember that infants with food-induced enterocolitis usually have negative skin tests and RAST. The positive predictive value of skin tests or RAST generally is less than 50%, although very high levels of food-specific IgE are as-

Table 3: Diagnosing Food Allergy

History

- Temporal association of symptoms with ingestion of a specific food
- Reproducible reactions each time the food protein is eaten
- Reaction involves typical organ systems (skin, gastrointestinal, respiratory)

Physical examination

- Signs of atopic disease
- Exclude other disorders

Laboratory

- Prick skin tests
- Radioallergosorbent test

Trial elimination diet

- Exclude suspect foods from diet for 1 to 2 weeks
- If results are not clear, consider food challenge

Food challenges

- Open challenge
- Double-blind, placebo-controlled food challenge
- Be prepared to treat possible adverse reactions

sociated with a greater risk of allergy.[21] Consequently, it is important to verify food allergies suspected on the basis of positive skin tests or RAST either with solid historical data or with food challenge procedures.

Eliminating suspect foods from the diet for 1 or 2 weeks may provide helpful information in some cases. A clear-cut improvement in symptoms suggests food allergy, but nega-

Table 4: Food Allergy Management Checklist

Exclude the offending food protein(s) from the diet

- Read food ingredient labels
- Carry pocket-sized reference cards
- Meet with schoolteachers or other caregivers of allergic children
- Take extra care when eating away from home
- Label hospital charts

Prescribe treatment for accidental ingestions

- Diphenhydramine 1 mg/kg/dose (50 mg maximum) orally, every 4-6 hours for reactions limited to the skin
- Epinephrine (1:1000) 0.01 mL/kg/dose (0.3 mL maximum) intramuscularly every 15-20 min for systemic or respiratory reactions
- If epinephrine is used, the patient should be transported to a medical facility ASAP
- Observe patient for at least 3-4 hours after accidental ingestion, and consider hospitalization for severe reactions

Consider purchasing a medical alert bracelet

Reevaluate patients every 1-3 years to determine if the allergy has resolved

- Exceptions: peanut, tree nut, fish, and shellfish allergies tend to be lifelong

Table 5: Recommended Dietary Allowances

Age	Calcium (mg)	Vitamin D (mg)
0-6 months	400	7.5
6-12 months	600	10
1-10 years	800	10
11-18 years	1,200	10

Committee on Dietary Allowances and Food and Nutrition Board, National Academy of Science, 1989;40:332.

tive or equivocal responses may require further evaluations because of the limitations inherent in compliance with dietary restrictions. If the elimination diet is being used as a diagnostic tool, the patient should return to clinic for follow-up in several weeks to ensure that the dietary restrictions do not become permanent without verification of food allergy.

Most cases of food allergy can be diagnosed on the basis of characteristic clinical manifestations that are temporarily associated with eating a particular food, detection of food-specific IgE, and improvement when the food is eliminated from the diet. Additional diagnostic studies may be needed in some cases, such as for unusual symptoms or for delayed reactions to food, or when allergy to multiple foods is suspected. Under these circumstances, food challenges are useful in verifying or disproving food allergies.[22,23] Challenge procedures can be performed using several formats: open, single-blind, or double-blind with a placebo control. Open challenges are particularly useful for quickly excluding food allergy in low-risk individuals, as in the case of a patient with negative skin tests. Because psychologic factors can strongly influence subjective reactions, blind challenges are helpful in many cases. Blinding the observer as

Table 6: Infant Formulas With Reduced Antigenicity

	Nutramigen®	Pregestamil®
Manufacturer	Mead Johnson (Princeton,NJ)	Mead Johnson
Protein source	Casein hydrolysate	Casein hydrolysate
Recommended for milk-allergic patients	Yes*	Yes*
Recommended for prevention of food allergy/AD	Yes	Yes
Comments		Fat source: medium-chain triglycerides

*Allergic reactions to formulas based on extensively hydrolyzed milk protein are rare but have been reported.

well allows for unbiased observations that have greater clinical validity. In setting up a double-blind, placebo-controlled food challenge, it is often useful to enlist the help of a dietitian who can prepare the challenge substances in a suitable vehicle to disguise their taste. The general principle behind food challenge is to initially administer a very low dose of the suspected allergen, then increase the dose at timed intervals until the subject has either eaten a typical portion of the food or shows manifestations of allergy.

Good Start®	Alimentum®	Neocate®
Nestle/ Carnation (Glendale, CA)	Ross Products/ Abbott Laboratories (Abbott Park, IL)	Scientific Hospital Supplies (Gaithersburg, MD)
Partial whey hydrolysate	Casein hydrolysate	Amino acids
No	Yes*	Yes
?	Yes	Yes
Commonly causes allergic symptoms in children with cow milk allergy		Amino acids are often tolerated by infants who have adverse reactions to hydrolyzed milk protein

Standards and safeguards for performing food challenges have been proposed.[22,23] Because severe reactions can occur even under controlled conditions, food challenges should only be performed at a medical facility where resuscitative equipment is available, such as epinephrine, respiratory support, and intravenous fluids. It is neither advisable nor necessary to conduct oral challenge tests on patients with a straightforward history of severe anaphylaxis and evidence of food-specific IgE.

Treatment of Food Allergy

The only treatment that has proven to be effective in food allergy is to completely exclude the offending food protein from the diet (Table 4).[6,8,10] Although this is simple in principle, accidental ingestion of allergenic foods is common, even among highly motivated patients.[24] Patients or parents must be taught to carefully read the labels of prepared foods and to recognize all forms of the allergenic protein. For example, casein, whey, and sodium caseinate are all forms of cow's milk protein. In addition, special precautions must be taken when eating away from home. Restaurant and school personnel often misunderstand food allergy or do not really know what is in the food they are serving. In two recent surveys of fatal or near-fatal food-induced anaphylaxis, eating away from home was identified as a major risk factor for unsuspected ingestion of a known allergen.[12,13] Parents sending children with food allergy to school or day care for the first time should meet with teachers or other caretakers to clearly explain dietary restrictions and contingency plans for the treatment of accidental ingestion of an allergen.[25]

Excluding one or two foods from the diet is unlikely to lead to nutritional deficiencies, with the possible exception of cow's milk allergy in an infant or young child. Milk is an important source of vitamin D and calcium, and supplements may be necessary to ensure that the recommended daily allowance of these nutrients is achieved (Table 5). Several infant formulas have been developed to have reduced antigenicity (Table 6).[26,27] Infants who are allergic to milk and soy usually do well when they are fed formulas that have either extensive hydrolyzed protein or amino acids as the protein source. It should be noted that Good Start® formula contains *partially* hydrolyzed milk protein and is not suitable for milk-allergic patients. Finally, patients who exclude multiple food proteins from their diet should be reevaluated because allergy to more than one or two foods is uncommon.[6,8,10]

Accidental ingestion of known food allergens is a common problem, and all patients with food allergy should be prepared for this possibility.[24] For reactions that are limited to the skin, a fast-acting antihistamine such as diphenhydramine (Benadryl®) or hydroxyzine (Atarax®, Vistaril®) should be administered (Table 4). For more serious reactions involving recurrent vomiting or evidence of respiratory or cardiovascular compromise, epinephrine should be administered immediately. Delaying the use of epinephrine may lead to more severe or even fatal reactions.[12,13] Patients with food allergy should routinely be prescribed epinephrine and should carry it with them at all times. Injectable epinephrine is available in several forms; however, the EpiPen® (0.3 mg) and EpiPen® Jr. (0.15 mg) are especially easy to use, which is a distinct advantage in an emergency. Medical alert bracelets are also recommended for patients who have experienced anaphylactic reactions in the past.

The Food Allergy & Anaphylaxis Network (10400 Eaton Place, Suite 107, Fairfax, VA 22030-2208, telephone 703-691-3179, homepage: http://www.foodallergy.org) is a support organization that was founded by parents of children with food allergy and is a valuable source of information, such as how to deal with schools, special recipes for food-allergic individuals, and pocket-sized guides to reading ingredient labels.

Natural History of Food Allergy

Most affected children eventually outgrow food allergy. Approximately one third of children and adults who are allergic to common allergens such as egg, milk, soy, and wheat lose their allergies 2 to 3 years after the initial diagnosis.[9,23] Most affected infants lose their food allergy by 3 years of age.[5] Children with food allergies should therefore be periodically reevaluated to see whether their allergies are still active. Unfortunately, allergies to peanuts, tree nuts, and seafood are unlikely to resolve and may be lifelong afflictions.[24,28]

Summary

Most food allergies are recognized and treated by primary health-care providers. Careful evaluation of the history and physical findings, performance of RAST or skin testing, and use of elimination diets provide sufficient information to evaluate many food-related complaints. Supplemental use of food challenge procedures is helpful in clarifying cases with lingering uncertainties. After food allergy is diagnosed, treatment is based on excluding the food allergen from the diet. It is essential to prepare patients with food allergy for accidental (and inevitable) ingestion of food allergens. Finally, it is important to realize that most children will eventually lose their food allergy; therefore, food allergy should be reevaluated periodically. Careful evaluation of food-related complaints results in accurate diagnosis of food allergies and the avoidance of unwarranted dietary restrictions and associated nutritional deficiencies.

References

1. Lake AM: Food protein-induced gastroenteropathy in infants and children. In: Metcalfe DD, Sampson HA, Simon RA, eds. *Food Allergy: Adverse Reactions to Foods and Food Additives*. Boston, Blackwell Scientific Publications, 1997, pp 277-286.

2. Godkin A, Tewell D: The pathogenesis of celiac disease. *Gastroenterology* 1998;115:206-210.

3. Sampson HA: Food allergy: part 1. Immunopathogenesis and clinical disorders. *J Allergy Clin Immunol* 1999;103:717-728.

4. Morrow JD, Margolies GR, Rowland J, et al: Evidence that histamine is the causative toxin of scombroid-fish poisoning. *N Engl J Med* 1991;324:716-720.

5. Bock SA: Prospective appraisal of complaints of adverse reactions to foods in children during the first 3 years of life. *Pediatrics* 1987;79:683-688.

6. Sampson HA: Food allergy. *JAMA* 1997;278:1888-1894.

7. David TJ, Waddington E, Stanton RH: Nutritional hazards of elimination diets in children with atopic eczema. *Arch Dis Child* 1984;59:323-325.

8. Bock SA, Atkins FM: Patterns of food hypersensitivity during sixteen years of double-blind, placebo-controlled food challenges. *J Pediatr* 1990;117:561-567.

9. Sampson HA, McCaskill CC: Food hypersensitivity and atopic dermatitis: evaluation of 113 patients. *J Pediatr* 1985;107: 669-675.

10. Goldman AS, Anderson DW, Sellers WA, et al: Milk allergy. I. Oral challenge with milk and isolated milk proteins in allergic children. *Pediatrics* 1963;32:425-443.

11. James JM, Bernhisel-Broadbent J, Sampson HA: Respiratory reactions provoked by double-blind food challenges in children. *Am J Respir Crit Care Med* 1994;149:59-64.

12. Sampson HA, Mendelson L, Rosen JP: Fatal and near-fatal anaphylactic reactions to food in children and adolescents *N Engl J Med* 1992;327:380-384.

13. Yuninger JW, Sweeney KG, Sturner WQ, et al: Fatal food-induced anaphylaxis. *JAMA* 1988;260:1450-1452.

14. Anderson JA: Mechanisms in adverse reactions to food. The brain. *Allergy* 1995;50:78-81.

15. Condemi JJ: Unproved diagnostic and therapeutic techniques. In: Metcalfe DD, Sampson HA, Simon RA, eds. *Food Allergy: Adverse Reactions to Foods and Food Additives*. Boston, Blackwell Scientific Publications, 1997, pp 541-550.

16. Ferguson A: Food sensitivity or self-deception? *N Engl J Med* 1990;323:476-478.

17. Pearson DJ, Rix KJ, Bentley SJ: Food allergy: how much in the mind? A clinical and psychiatric study of suspected food hypersensitivity. *Lancet* 1983;1:1259-1261.

18. Powell GK: Milk- and soy- induced enterocolitis of infancy. Clinical features and standardization of challenge. *J Pediatr* 1978;93:553-560.

19. Burks AW, Sampson HA: Diagnostic approaches to the patient with suspected food allergies. *J Pediatr* 1992;121:S64-S71.

20. Yuninger JW, Ahlstedt S, Eggleston PA, et al: Quantitative IgE antibody assays in allergic diseases. *J Allergy Clin Immunol* 2000;105:1077-1084.

21. Sampson HA, Ho DG: Relationship between food-specific IgE concentrations and the risk of positive food challenges in children and adolescents. *J Allergy Clin Immunol* 1997;100:444-451.

22. Niggemann B, Wahn U, Sampson HA: Proposals for standardization of oral food challenge tests in infants and children. *Pediatr Allergy Immunol* 1994;5:11-13.

23. Bock SA, Sampson HA, Atkins FM, et al: Double-blind, placebo-controlled food challenge (DBPCFC) as an office procedure: a manual. *J Allergy Clin Immunol* 1988;82:986-997.

24. Bock SA, Atkins FM: The natural history of peanut allergy. *J Allergy Clin Immunol* 1989;83:900-904.

25. Frazier CA, Wynn SR, Munoz-Furlong A, et al: Anaphylaxis at school: etiologic factors, prevalence, and treatment. *Pediatrics* 1993;91:516.

26. Gern JE, Lemanske RF: Pediatric allergy: can it be prevented? *Immunol Allergy Clin North Am* 1999;19:233-252.

27. American Academy of Pediatrics, Committee on Nutrition: Hypoallergenic infant formulas. *Pediatrics* 2000;106:346-349.

28. Daul CB, Morgan JE Lehrer SB: The natural history of shrimp hypersensitivity. *J Allergy Clin Immunol* 1990;86:88-93.

12

Iatrogenic Allergies: Drugs and Latex

Adverse reactions to medications are among the most common problems encountered by health-care providers. Such drug reactions occur in 2% to 3% of hospitalized patients[1] and in a sizable proportion of outpatients who are treated with a variety of medications. When evaluating an adverse reaction to a medicine, it is important to distinguish allergic reactions that have an immunologic basis from reactions triggered by other causes, such as drug intolerance, pharmacologic side effects, or idiosyncratic reactions. Examples of drug side effects that are not allergic in nature arc abdominal pain secondary to erythromycin and albuterol-induced tremor. In most instances, a careful review of the history and the physical findings is sufficient to distinguish drug allergies from other reactions, but in some cases skin testing or in vitro testing for drug-specific immunoglobulin E (IgE) can provide definitive information.

Clinical Manifestations and Mechanisms of Adverse Drug Reactions

Immunologic reactions to drugs or latex can occur via several different mechanisms. The timing of an allergic reaction after a drug administration and the organ systems that are affected are important clues to the relevant patho-

Table 1: Clinical Manifestations of Immediate Drug Hypersensitivity

Organ system	Signs and symptoms
Skin	Urticaria
	Angioedema
	Flushing
	Pruritus
Gastrointestinal	Oral pruritus
	Vomiting
	Abdominal pain
	Diarrhea
Respiratory	Rhinorrhea
	Tearing
	Wheezing
	Laryngeal edema
Neurologic	Obtundation
	Loss of consciousness
Cardiovascular	Tachycardia
	Hypotension

genic mechanism and have significant diagnostic and therapeutic implications. Reactions that occur rapidly after the first or second dose of a medicine are likely to be caused by immediate or type I hypersensitivity, which involves the activation of mast cells and subsequent release of noxious mediators such as histamine and leukotrienes (see Chapter 2). Once released, mast cell mediators rapidly induce allergic signs and symptoms. Therefore, mast cell mediated allergic reactions to intravenous or inhaled allergens usually begin within minutes of allergen exposure. Reactions that follow oral medications are sometimes delayed by 1 to 2 hours, probably because of the time required to absorb the allergen. Immediate hypersensitivity reactions can involve several organ systems, including the skin, gastrointestinal tract, respiratory system, cardiovascular system, and central nervous system (Table 1).

Mast cells can be triggered via several different pathways, including the cross-linking of surface IgE, the generation of anaphylatoxins (C3a, C5a), or the direct effects of a drug on mediator release. Many low-molecular-weight drugs (eg, penicillin) act as haptens and must first bind to a carrier protein to form a complex large enough to cross-link IgE and trigger the mast cell. In contrast, some drugs trigger mast cell mediator release directly, and this produces clinical findings that are indistinguishable from IgE-mediated allergy.[2] These reactions are called anaphylactoid reactions and are most commonly triggered by codeine and other opiates, by intravenous contrast dye, and by protamine.

Nonsteroidal anti-inflammatory drugs, such as aspirin, produce adverse reactions in a subset of patients through pharmacologic effects on prostaglandin and leukotriene metabolism.[3] In these individuals, aspirin or related drugs cause overproduction of leukotrienes and mast cell activation, through mechanisms that have not been clearly defined. Finally, intravenous infusion of γ-globulin can cause immediate reactions that occur through an immune complex mediated mechanism. During rapid infusion of intravenous γ-globulin, small amounts of immune complexes present in the preparation can activate complement, causing fever, chills, skin rashes, and sometimes hypotension.

In contrast to immediate hypersensitivity reactions, some responses appear days or weeks after the initiation of therapy. Serum sickness, which is the most common form of delayed drug reaction, was first described in the early 1900s in patients who were treated with infusions of horse serum for various infectious diseases. Similar reactions have been observed in recent years after administration of antithymocyte globulin (also derived from horse serum), which is used in preparative regimens before transplantation.[4] The mechanism of serum sickness is related to the production of drug-specific IgM and IgE antibodies. After 7 to 10 days of drug administration, the antibodies reach concentrations similar to that of the drug, leading to the formation of immune complexes that subsequently activate complement and other inflammatory cascades. Clinical manifestations usually begin insidiously,[4] and recognition of early signs and symptoms requires a high index of suspicion. Skin manifestations vary and include urticaria, erythema multiforme, and vasculitic rashes. Systemic manifestations of serum sickness reactions include fever, myalgia, abdominal pain, and generalized malaise. Joint swelling, liver inflammation, and eosinophilia also frequently occur. If these reactions are not recognized at an early stage, severe dermatitis and mucosal desquamation (Stevens-Johnson syndrome) can develop. Sulfisoxazole (Gantrisin®, Pediazole®), phenytoin (Dilantin®), cefaclor (Ceclor®), and penicillin are the medications most commonly associated with serum sickness reactions.

Drug reactions produced by delayed-type hypersensitivity (type IV) reactions are usually limited to the skin or conjunctiva. An example is a skin rash that occurs 1 to 2 days after starting treatment with a topical eye drop or ointment. This type of reaction requires prior sensitization, during which drug-specific CD4+ T cells were stimulated.[5] Within 48 hours of reexposure, antigen-specific T cells home to the area of exposure and orchestrate local inflammation, which can be intense. The hallmark of the resulting contact dermatitis is that skin findings, which usually include redness, pruritus, and dermal edema or vesiculation, are usually sharply demarcated and correspond to the area to which the medication was applied.[6,7]

Medications can also trigger anemia, thrombocytopenia, or neutropenia by binding to cellular proteins and setting off an autoimmune reaction. For example, penicillin can initiate type II hypersensitivity reactions by binding to the surface of red blood cells, creating a 'neoantigen' that is recognized by circulating antibodies, leading to activation of complement and phagocytic cells.[8]

Skin Testing in the Clinical Evaluation of Drug Allergy

Immediate hypersensitivity skin tests or radioallergosorbent test (RAST) should only be considered when the history and clinical findings are compatible with a type I reaction. Reliable skin test reagents are available only for penicillin and penicillin derivatives. Skin testing protocols to detect allergy to other medications, including sulfa, insulin, and local anesthetics, have been published, but relatively little data exist regarding their sensitivity or specificity.

Skin testing for penicillin allergy is highly predictive of future reactions to penicillin and related medications.[9,10] However, skin tests that are negative for penicillin do not exclude the possibility of cephalosporin allergy.[11] The results of a penicillin skin test reflect the current state of sensitization and do not predict whether the patient will become resensitized in the future after additional courses of penicillin. Patients who have a history of hypersensitivity reactions to penicillin but have negative penicillin skin tests have only a 1% to 3% chance of developing a urticarial reaction during penicillin therapy. This risk is similar to that of the general population.[1,10] The risk of an anaphylactic reaction to penicillin following negative skin tests is approximately 1 in 1,000.[1,10] On the other hand, patients with a history of penicillin hypersensitivity who have positive skin tests have a 50% to 60% chance of developing a systemic reaction after penicillin administration.[1,10]

Patch testing can be helpful in identifying the offending medication in cases of drug-induced contact dermatitis, although the diagnosis is often made on clinical grounds. However, if preparations with many ingredients have been applied to the skin and if identity of the allergen is unclear, it is important to positively identify the allergen to avoid future problems. Despite recent advances in the standardization of allergen preparations and techniques,[6,12] there are many causes of false-positive and false-negative results.[13] This problem is even more evident when testing with materials that have not been standardized, which is often necessary because of the limited number of commercially available standardized extracts. Thus, patch testing should be performed only by physicians who have been formally trained in this technique.

Treatment of Allergic Reactions to Drugs

Managing allergic reactions to drugs involves five principles: (1) identifying the relevant mechanism; (2) identifying the drug causing the reaction; (3) deciding whether to discontinue the medication; (4) providing supportive care to involve medical therapy for anaphylactic-type symptoms as well as less severe reactions such as urticaria; and (5) consideration of desensitization therapy. The decision whether to stop treatment with a particular medication or to continue treatment in the face of a drug reaction depends on several factors. In most instances, it is best to discontinue a medication that is causing an allergic reaction, but sometimes it is in a patient's best interest to continue the offending medication while carefully monitoring the course of a mild allergic reaction, such as intermittent urticaria. In the case of a severe allergic reaction, the offending drug should be discontinued unless there is a compelling reason not to do so. However, if erythema multiforme or mucosal involvement is present, then the offending medication should be stopped immediately to minimize the chances of Stevens-Johnson syndrome, a potentially life-threatening disorder.

If a drug with similar pharmacologic effects will be substituted, the clinician should avoid using antigenically similar drugs (eg, erythromycin, clarithromycin [Biaxin®]) because of cross-reactivity. If a patient has a penicillin allergy, it is best to avoid use of all medications that share the basic penicillin backbone, including semisynthetic penicillins, some cephalosporins, and imipenem. Aztreonam (Azactam®), a monobactam, has negligible cross-reactivity with penicillin and can thus be used with a high degree of safety in penicillin-allergic patients.[14] The newer cephalosporins, which are distinct from penicillin, can also be used safely in most patients with penicillin allergy.[15]

Anaphylactic reactions to medications should be treated as outlined in Chapter 14. Reactions that are limited to the skin often respond to the use of antihistamines to relieve itching or urticaria. Drug-induced urticaria can last several weeks even after the offending medication has been discontinued. Manifestations of serum sickness-type reactions, such as myalgia and joint swelling, are treated with nonsteroidal anti-inflammatory medications or, in severe cases, with oral corticosteroids.

Preventive measures to reduce the chances for future allergic reactions include desensitization, prophylactic use of medications before anticipated exposure to allergens, and communicating information about a patient's drug allergies to all members of the health-care team. Desensitization regimens are effective for treating allergy to several medications, including sulfa, penicillin, and aspirin.[1,16,17] Desensitization is best achieved via the oral route, which is as effective as parenteral desensitization but is associated with a lower incidence of anaphylaxis.[1] Desensitization should only be performed under close observation, such as in a hospital ward that allows for cardiac monitoring of the patient and that is fully equipped to treat anaphylaxis. Table 2 depicts a standard oral desensitization regimen for penicillin.[1]

In patients with a known hypersensitivity to intravenous radiocontrast material, premedication regimens may decrease, but not necessarily eliminate, the frequency or the severity of allergic reactions. These regimens include pretreatment with antihistamines and corticosteroids (see Chapter 14). The use of a nonionic radiocontrast material should also be considered in high-risk individuals.[18,19] Finally, flagging the patient's medical record and notifying inpatient or outpatient pharmacies of drug reactions are important precautionary measures. Medical alert bracelets or necklaces may be appropriate for patients with particularly severe allergies.

Table 2: Oral Desensitization Regimen for β-Lactam Medications*

Step (15-min intervals)	Drug concentration (mg/mL)
1	0.5
2	0.5
3	0.5
4	0.5
5	0.5
6	0.5
7	0.5
8	5
9	5
10	5
11	50
12	50
13	50
14	50

After step 14, observe the patient for 30 minutes. If there is no adverse reaction, administer 1 g of the same agent intravenously.

Latex Allergy

Although contact sensitivity to natural rubber or latex has been recognized for more than a century, IgE-mediated reactions to latex have only been widely recognized in the past decade. The reason for the recent surge in the incidence of allergy to natural rubber is unknown but is proba-

Volume** (mL)	Dose given (mg)	Cumulative dose (mg)
0.1	0.05	0.05
0.2	0.1	0.15
0.4	0.2	0.35
0.8	0.4	0.75
1.6	0.8	1.6
3.2	1.6	3.2
6.4	3.2	6.4
1.2	6	12
2.4	12	24
4.8	24	48
1	50	98
2	100	198
4	200	398
8	400	798

* Modified from Sullivan,[1] used with permission.
** Dilute the drug suspension into 30 mL water for ingestion.

bly related to the widespread use of latex gloves in the hospital as part of universal precautions to inhibit the spread of infectious diseases. Certain groups are at much higher risk for latex allergy than the general population[20] and are listed in Table 3. The common factor uniting these groups is increased exposure to natural rubber products, either in the

Table 3: Risk Factors for Latex Allergy

- Spina bifida
- Urologic abnormalities
- Health-care workers
- Latex industry workers
- Food allergy
- Repeated surgeries
- Unexplained intraoperative anaphylaxis

health-care setting or in the workplace. In some groups, such as individuals with spina bifida or those with urologic abnormalities who have required several surgeries, the risk of latex sensitivity is high enough to warrant latex avoidance precautions even in the absence of signs or symptoms of latex allergy.[21]

Clinical manifestations of latex allergy depend on the mechanism of the immunologic reaction.[20] Signs and symptoms of latex-induced contact dermatitis, which is a type IV reaction mediated by sensitized T cells, are limited to the skin. These include redness, itching, and edema, accompanied by vesiculation and, occasionally, localized urticaria. The skin rash typically follows exposure to latex within 24 to 72 hours, although the temporal relationship may be obscured if exposure to latex is chronic. IgE-mediated latex reactions, on the other hand, are characterized by skin, respiratory, and systemic manifestations typical of type I allergy. It is important to realize that some patients may become exquisitely sensitive to latex proteins and develop symptoms when exposed to minute amounts of latex, such as airborne dust particles from gloves that are opened in the same room as the patient.[22] Also, several foods contain proteins that cross-react with latex allergens and can provoke allergic reactions in latex-allergic

Table 4: Latex Exposure in the Home and Office

- Balloons
- Adhesive tape
- Elastic bands in clothing
- Rubber erasers
- Sports balls
- Carpet backing
- Rubber bands
- Rubber trees

Note: 'Latex' paint is actually made of acrylic instead of natural rubber and does not pose a threat to latex-allergic patients.

patients. These foods include bananas, avocados, cherries, plums, and chestnuts.[21,23]

The diagnosis of latex allergy is often clinically obvious, because exposure to latex is common in the home, at work, and in health-care environments. Skin tests or RAST can be used to verify the presence of latex-specific IgE, which strongly supports the diagnosis of type I latex allergy.[23] This can also be helpful in evaluating whether urticaria secondary to latex exposure is from contact dermatitis or from IgE-mediated allergy. A latex-specific RAST is available in the United States, but negative results should be interpreted with caution because up to 25% of all patients with proven latex allergy may have negative RAST results.[24] A latex antigen extract is being developed, and a multicenter clinical trial found that this skin test reagent had a high degree of safety and diagnostic accuracy.[25] Pending approval of a standardized test, skin testing may be performed using unstandardized latex extracts, which are prepared by soaking cut-up glove fragments in diluent. However, the concentration of latex proteins in such preparations varies considerably. In addition, systemic reactions to latex skin testing can occur,[26] and thus skin testing with latex should not be performed in patients who are suspected of being exquisitely sensitive to latex.

Table 5: Latex Exposure in the Clinic and Hospital

Items containing latex	Latex-free replacements*
Adhesive tape, bandage strips	Paper tape, plastic tape, silk tape
Latex gloves	Gloves made of vinyl, nitrile, neoprene, or other synthetic materials
Urologic catheters	Silicone or plastic catheters
Stethoscope tubing	Plastic tubing
Tourniquets	Plastic tourniquets (or apply tourniquet over clothing)
Blood pressure cuffs	Plastic cuff (or apply cuff over clothing)
Ambu bag	Silicone or vinyl bags, masks, and reservoirs
Syringes	Glass syringes
Injection ports	Flush tubing and cover latex ports (use stopcock to infuse medications)
Medication vial stoppers	Single-use glass ampules

* Always check with the manufacturer or supplier to determine whether an individual product contains latex.

The only proven therapy for latex allergy is avoidance. Because latex-derived products are ubiquitous in modern society (Table 4), this requires a dedicated effort. In addition, hospital and clinic staff should prepare protocols to ensure the safety of latex-allergic patients.[21] This should include having on hand supplies of latex-free materials such as gloves, urologic catheters, and tourniquets (Table 5). The Spina Bifida Association of America (4590 MacArthur Boulevard NW, Suite 250, Washington, DC 20007; 800-621-3141, http://www.sbaa.org) is an excellent source of information about latex-free medical supplies.

As with drug allergy, it is critically important to indicate in the hospital and clinic that the patient is latex allergic to avoid inadvertent exposure. This can be achieved by posting 'latex allergy' signs and stickers on the patient's hospital room, door, bed, and charts. Maintaining a latex-safe environment for an inpatient can be difficult, given the many people who enter the typical hospital room during any 24-hour period, and can only be accomplished by careful planning and staff education. Perhaps the most effective means of reducing exposure in the medical environment is to gradually replace latex-containing materials with nonlatex substitutes. In addition, it has recently been proposed that powdered latex gloves be replaced with either nonlatex gloves or powder-free low-protein latex gloves, which shed much less allergen into the environment.

It is especially challenging to provide a latex-safe environment in the operating room. Many hospitals have set aside one hospital operating room in which no latex-containing equipment or supplies are used. In addition, patients who are scheduled for the operating room can be started on a prophylactic regimen of antihistamines and corticosteroids similar to that used in patients with type IV radiocontrast hypersensitivity (Chapter 14), although this regimen has not yet been evaluated in controlled trials.

References

1. Sullivan TJ: Drug allergy. In: Middleton E Jr, Reed CE, Ellis EF, et al, eds. *Allergy: Principles and Practice*. St. Louis, Mosby-Year Book, 1993, pp 1726-1746.

2. VanArsdel PP Jr: Pseudoallergic drug reactions. *Immunol Allergy Clin North Am* 1991;11:635-644.

3. Israel E, Fischer AR, Rosenberg MA, et al: The pivotal role of 5-lipoxygenase products in the reaction of aspirin-sensitive asthmatics to aspirin. *Am Rev Respir Dis* 1993;148:1447-1451.

4. Lawley TJ, Bielory L, Gascon P, et al: A prospective clinical and immunologic analysis of patients with serum sickness. *N Engl J Med* 1984;311:1407-1413.

5. Wood GS, Volterra AS, Abel EA, et al: Allergic contact dermatitis: novel immunohistologic features. *J Invest Dermatol* 1986; 87:688-693.

6. Rietschel RL: Occupational contact dermatitis. *Lancet* 1997;349: 1093-1095.

7. Klaus MV, Wieselthier JS: Contact dermatitis. *Am Fam Physician* 1993;48:629-632.

8. Dove AF, Thomas DJ, Aronstam A, et al: Haemolytic anaemia due to penicillin. *Br Med J* 1975;3:684.

9. Sogn DD, Evans R 3d, Shepherd GM, et al: Results of the National Institute of Allergy and Infectious Diseases Collaborative Clinical Trial to test the predictive value of skin testing with major and minor penicillin derivatives in hospitalized adults. *Arch Intern Med* 1992;152:1025-1032.

10. Pichichero ME, Pichichero DM: Diagnosis of penicillin, amoxicillin, and cephalosporin allergy: reliability of examination assessed by skin testing and oral challenge. *J Pediatr* 1998;132:137-143.

11. Romano A, Mayorga C, Torres MJ, et al: Immediate allergic reactions to cephalosporins: cross reactivity and selected responses. *J Allergy Clin Immunol* 2000;106:1177-1183.

12. Brasch J, Henseler T, Aberer W, et al: Reproducibility of patch tests. A multicenter study of synchronous left- versus right-sided patch tests by the German Contact Dermatitis Research Group. *J Am Acad Dermatol* 1994;31:584-591.

13. Oshima H, Kawahara D, Hashimoto Y, et al: An approach to evaluating patch test results. *Contact Dermatitis* 1994;31:189-191.

14. Moss RB: Sensitization to aztreonam and cross-reactivity with other beta-lactam antibiotics in high-risk patients with cystic fibrosis. *J Allergy Clin Immunol* 1991;87:78-88.

15. Anne S, Reisman RE: Risk of administering cephalosporin antibiotics to patients with histories of penicillin allergy. *Ann Allergy Asthma Immunol* 1995;74:167-170.

16. Kletzel M, Beck S, Elser J, et al: Trimethoprim-sulfamethoxazole oral desensitization in hemophiliacs infected with human immunodeficiency virus with a history of hypersensitivity reactions. *Am J Dis Child* 1991;145:1428-1429.

17. Bush RK, Asbury D: Aspirin-sensitive asthma. In: Busse WW, Holgate ST, eds. *Asthma and Rhinitis*. Boston, Blackwell Scientific Publications, 1995, pp 1429-1439.

18. Cohan RH, Dunnick NR, Bashore TM: Treatment of reactions to radiographic contrast material. *AJR Am J Roentgenol* 1988;151:263-270.

19. Bush WH, Swanson DP: Radiocontrast. In: Virant SL, ed. *Systemic Reactions*. Philadelphia, WB Saunders, 1995, pp 597-612.

20. Poley GE, Slater JE: Latex allergy. *J Allergy Clin Immunol* 2000;105:1054-1062.

21. Kelly KJ: Management of the latex-allergic patient. *Immunol Allergy Clin North Am* 1995;15:139-157.

22. Sussman GL, Tarlo S, Dolovich J: The spectrum of IgE-mediated responses to latex. *JAMA* 1991;265:2844-2847.

23. Granady LC, Slater JE: The history and diagnosis of latex allergy. *Immunol Allergy Clin North Am* 1995;15:21-29.

24. Hamilton RG, et al: Diagnostic performance of Food and Drug Administration-cleared serologic assays for natural rubber latex-specific IgE antibody. *J Allergy Clin Immunol* 1999; 103:925-930.

25. Spaner D, Dolovich J, Tarlo S, et al: Hypersensitivity to natural latex. *J Allergy Clin Immunol* 1989;83:1135-1137.

26. Hamilton RG, et al: Diagnosis of natural rubber latex allergy: multicenter latex skin testing efficacy study. *J Allergy Clin Immunol* 1998;102:482-490.

13

Diagnosis and Treatment of Insect Sting Allergy

Most allergic reactions associated with insect stings are caused by members of the Hymenoptera order, which includes bees, wasps, hornets, yellow jackets, and fire ants. The offending insects vary with geographic location: in the United States, yellow jackets account for most allergic reactions, while in Europe, more than 95% of insect sting reactions are caused by honeybees and wasps.[1] Allergic reactions to fire ants are becoming more common in the southern United States, coinciding with expansion of that insect's habitat northward from Central America and Mexico. Allergic reactions can also be triggered by insects that bite rather than sting their victims.[2] However, allergic reactions to biting insects, which include mosquitoes, horse flies, deer flies, and fleas, are relatively uncommon and will not be examined in this chapter.

When evaluating allergic reactions, medical personnel should have a basic understanding of the life cycle of stinging insects.[2,3] Because yellow jackets nest in the ground, they often sting victims who are mowing the lawn or walking barefoot outdoors. These insects are attracted by food and beverages such as meat, fish, fruit juices, colas, and beer. It is common to encounter swarms of yellow jackets around garbage or compost receptacles. Yellow jackets are aggressive and often sting even if unprovoked. Bumblebees also nest in the ground but are relatively docile. In general, bumblebees and honeybees sting only if their nests are disturbed or if they are trapped inside clothes. The exception is the Africanized bee, or so-called killer bee, which is more aggressive than domestic bees. These insects have spread from Mexico into Texas and other parts of the Southwest, where cases involving multiple stings are becoming more common. Wasps and hornets typically nest well above the ground, so it is unusual for stings to occur unless the nest is disturbed. One difference between these insects and the honeybee is that wasps and hornets can inflict multiple stings. Finally, the fire ant is found mainly in the southern United States.[4] Nests can be recognized by their low hills with multiple entrances. The hallmark of the fire ant sting is the appearance of a sterile pustule within 24 hours.

Adverse Reactions to Insect Stings

Adverse reactions to insect stings can be classified as toxic reactions, large local reactions, urticarial reactions, and anaphylaxis. Each of these reactions typically appears a few minutes to several hours after the insect sting. Reactions that occur many hours after an insect sting are reported less commonly.[5] The pathogenesis for these late-onset reactions has not clearly been established.

Toxic reactions

Toxic reactions only occur after multiple stings and are caused by pharmacologic effects of the cumulative dose of venom.[2,3] Clinical manifestations of toxic reactions can closely resemble anaphylactic reactions, so they may be difficult to distinguish clinically. If there is doubt about the nature of the reaction, skin testing or radioallergosorbent test (RAST) can be used after the patient has recovered to help establish the diagnosis and to determine if desensitization therapy is warranted.

Large local reactions

Large local reactions that occur as the result of insect sting include localized swelling, itching, and pain that may begin minutes to hours after the sting. Peak symptoms usually occur within several days, and the swelling may persist for up to a week. Although large local reactions are uncomfortable, they are not dangerous. Furthermore, patients who have experienced local reactions are unlikely to develop more severe reactions after future insect stings.[6] For this reason, skin testing and desensitization therapy are not warranted after a large local reaction. The pathogenesis of these reactions is not known but may involve immunoglobulin E (IgE) antibodies in some cases. Treatment of large local reactions consists of providing symptomatic relief: cold compresses, nonsteroidal anti-inflammatory drugs, and antihistamines can all help relieve associated symptoms.

Generalized urticarial reactions

One of the more common adverse reactions to insect stings is urticaria, which can be either generalized or confined to the region surrounding the sting. The natural history of generalized urticarial reactions has been evaluated in a study of 242 children, including 86 children who did not receive immunotherapy.[7] In 196 repeat stings, only 9.2% of children developed systemic reactions, and none of these reactions was more severe than the original episode of generalized urticaria. Similar data are beginning to accumulate for adults with generalized dermal reactions after insect stings,[1,8] although definitive studies have not been completed. For now, it is recommended that adults with generalized urticaria undergo skin testing and be considered for venom immunotherapy.

Anaphylaxis

The estimated incidence of insect sting anaphylaxis in the general population is 0.3% to 3%.[3] Considering that these reactions can be fatal, it is surprising that nearly 50% of people with insect sting hypersensitivity never seek help for this problem. This is especially tragic considering that venom immunotherapy is highly effective for lowering the risk for subsequent anaphylactic reactions. Anaphylactic reactions occur most often in people under the age of 20; however, anaphylactic reactions are more likely to be fatal in the elderly. Another factor that increases the risk of fatality from an insect sting is the use of β-blocker medications such as propranolol (Inderal®).[9]

Virtually everyone is at risk for anaphylactic reactions from insect stings, but only one third of people with a history of insect sting-induced reactions have a history of allergy, and atopic individuals are not at increased risk for stinging insect allergy.[10] Several studies have been conducted to determine the natural history of severe insect sting hypersensitivity. In the United States, individuals who experience a sting-related anaphylactic reaction have a 50% to 60% risk for anaphylaxis after subsequent insect stings,[3] while studies performed in Europe suggest that the risk is approximately 30%.[11]

Anaphylaxis triggered by insect stings produces the same clinical manifestations found in anaphylaxis from other triggers (see Chapter 14). Signs and symptoms usually occur within minutes of the sting and include urticaria, angioedema, bronchospasm, laryngospasm, abdominal pain, tachycardia, hypotension, and loss of consciousness.[12]

Testing for Insect Sting Hypersensitivity

Skin testing is the preferred method for confirming the diagnosis of insect sting hypersensitivity,[13,14] but it should only be performed on those patients who are candidates for venom desensitization (Table 1).[2,3,7,15] These include adults or children with a history of anaphylactic reactions to insect stings or adults with generalized urticarial reactions. Toxic reactions, large local reactions, and generalized urticarial reactions in children do not warrant skin testing because the results would not alter the subsequent treatment. Standardized venom preparations are now available for all of the major members of the Hymenoptera order, including

Table 1: Insect Sting Reaction

Type of reaction	Mechanism	Skin testing indicated?
Toxic	Pharmacologic effects of venom	No
Large local	Local inflammation	No
Urticaria	IgE-mediated or complement activation	Adults - yes Children - no
Anaphylaxis	IgE-mediated	Yes

*If skin tests are positive
NSAID = nonsteroidal anti-inflammatory drug

yellow jackets, honeybees, white-faced hornets, wasps, and fire ants. Immediate skin test reactions to insect venoms at the concentration of 1.0 μg/mL or less indicate the presence of venom-specific IgE, although nonspecific reactions can occur with with venom concentrations of 1.0 μg/mL.[13]

Extensive cross-reactivity exists among the major allergens in the Hymenoptera order, especially among the vespids (yellow jackets, hornets, and wasps). Therefore, it is common to develop positive skin tests to multiple venoms after having an allergic reaction to a single vespid. Venom-specific RAST inhibition tests can positively identify a specific venom allergy in about half of cases in which there are multiple positive skin tests and the identity of the insect is unclear.[16] In RAST inhibition, purified venom extracts are used to inhibit binding of patient serum to a second venom allergen bound to a solid-phase substrate. In-

Acute therapy	Immunotherapy indicated?
Supportive	No
Cool packs, NSAIDs, antihistamines	No
Antihistamine, close observation	Adults - yes* Children - no
Epinephrine sub-Q, other resuscitation as needed	Yes*

complete inhibition indicates cross-reactivity. When the insect cannot be positively identified and there are multiple positive skin tests, immunotherapy with mixed venom preparations is recommended.

Venom-specific RASTs can be used in place of skin tests, although they are somewhat less sensitive.[13,17] Indications for using a RAST would include daily use of β-blockers, dermatographism, or generalized skin disease that precludes skin testing. A RAST is also an acceptable alternative if access to reliable skin testing is not available or if there is a strong clinical suspicion of venom allergy in a patient with negative skin tests.

Therapy

Treatment of insect stings depends on the nature and severity of the reaction. Most stings need no specific treatment, but significant local or systemic reactions may require acute medical management as well as preventive measures to decrease the chances of future reactions (Table 2).

Treatment of acute symptoms

Allergic reactions to insect stings should be treated in the same fashion as allergic reactions caused by other triggers.[2,3,15] Generalized reactions that are limited to skin should be treated with oral antihistamines such as diphenhydramine (Benadryl®, 1 mg/kg/dose q 6 h for children, 25 to 50 mg PO q 6 h for adults). If the reaction includes extracutaneous allergic manifestations, then subcutaneous epinephrine (1:1,000; 0.01 mL/kg for children, 0.3 to 0.5 mL for adults) should be administered. Remember that epinephrine (EpiPen®, Ana-Kit®) has a short half-life, and the dose may need to be repeated every 15 to 30 minutes. Patients who do not promptly and completely respond to 1 or 2 doses of epinephrine require insertion of a large-gauge intravenous catheter and prompt resuscitation with intravenous fluids (other measures are reviewed in Chapter 14). Patients who present with particularly severe reactions or those with protracted symptoms should be hospitalized because they are at increased risk for recurrent symptoms.

Preventive measures

Several common-sense precautions are available to people who have had an adverse reaction to insect stings, regardless of whether the reactions are IgE-mediated (Table 2). Most unprovoked stings are from yellow jackets, but the risk of being stung by these insects can be diminished by avoiding eating or drinking outdoors during the yellow jacket season. These insects congregate around compost or garbage, so it is best to keep these items separated as far as possible from living quarters. Fishermen are at especially high risk for yellow jacket stings because these insects are attracted by fish. Other precautions include wearing shoes, long-sleeved shirts, and pants outdoors and avoiding wearing clothes with floral colors.

Table 2: Overview of Therapy for Stinging Insect Allergy

Medical therapy for acute symptoms

Avoidance measures

- Avoid outdoor eating or drinking
- Wear shoes outdoors
- Wear long pants and long-sleeved shirts
- Avoid wearing perfume or cologne
- Avoid wearing floral-colored clothing
- Keep garbage or compost far away from living areas

Immunotherapy

Medical alert bracelets

Epinephrine for self-administration

- EpiPen®
- Ana-Kit®

People at risk for repeated occurrences of anaphylaxis, such as those who are just starting venom immunotherapy or those who refuse venom therapy, should carry epinephrine in a self-administered form. It is also important to prescribe epinephrine to patients who have had systemic reactions to insect stings and who are awaiting an allergic evaluation. Two commonly used devices are the Ana-Kit® (Hollister-Stier Laboratories, Spokane, WA) and the EpiPen® (Center Laboratories, Port Washington, NY). The EpiPen® is especially easy to use because it comes in a spring-loaded kit that can be administered through clothes. The Ana-Kit® has the advantage of providing more than one dose of epinephrine, but it requires more attention to technique, which can be a disadvantage in an emergency.

Venom Immunotherapy

Venom immunotherapy is essentially curative for the treatment of anaphylactic reactions to insect stings.[18,19] Patients who are candidates for venom immunotherapy include those with anaphylactic reactions as well as adults who have had generalized urticarial reactions. Immunotherapy involves injecting gradually increasing amounts of purified insect venom or, in the case of the fire ant, whole body extracts, to alter the immune response. Although the precise mechanism for venom immunotherapy is unknown, clinical protection is associated with increases in venom-specific IgG and decreases in venom-specific IgE.[19,20] It is debatable whether there is clinical merit in measuring either of these parameters in people who are undergoing venom immunotherapy.

Venom immunotherapy can be administered according to standard protocols that take 2 to 3 months to reach a maintenance dose or as a rush immunotherapy schedule that is especially helpful for fishermen and beekeepers, for whom resting is extremely likely.[21] Regardless of the schedule, once maintenance doses have been achieved, immunotherapy is usually continued monthly for an extended period of time. The optimum duration for immunotherapy has been the subject of much debate, but most allergists agree that a 3-year to 5-year treatment regimen is sufficient to produce permanent desensitization in many cases.[2,3,13,22] Longer courses of immunotherapy may be appropriate for people who have had more severe anaphylactic reactions.[23] Repeating venom skin tests can be helpful in deciding when to stop immunotherapy.

Summary

Insect sting hypersensitivity is a common clinical problem. Primary health-care providers can treat most sting symptoms by administering symptomatic relief and by advising patients how to avoid stings in the future. For severe reactions, including anaphylaxis and generalized urticarial reactions in adults, referral to an allergist is recommended, especially because venom immunotherapy is effective in preventing future episodes of anaphylaxis.

References

1. Muller UR: Epidemiology of insect sting allergy. *Monogr Allergy* 1993;31:131-146.

2. Yunginger JW: Insect allergy. In: Middleton E Jr, Reed CE, Ellis EF, et al, eds. *Allergy: Principles and Practice*. St. Louis, Mosby-Year Book, 1998, pp 1063-1072.

3. Reisman R: Insect stings. *N Engl J Med* 1994;331:523-527.

4. Freeman TM: Imported fire ants: the ants from hell! *Allergy Proc* 1994;15:11-15.

5. Reisman RE, Livingston A: Late-onset allergic reactions, including serum sickness, after insect stings. *J Allergy Clin Immunol* 1989;84:331-337.

6. Mauriello PM, Barde SH, Georgitis JW, et al: Natural history of large local reactions from stinging insects. *J Allergy Clin Immunol* 1984;74:494-498.

7. Valentine MD, Schuberth KC, Kagey-Sobotka A, et al: The value of immunotherapy with venom in children with allergy to insect stings. *N Engl J Med* 1990;323:1601-1603.

8. Reisman RE: Natural history of insect sting allergy: relationship of severity of symptoms of initial sting anaphylaxis to resting reactions. *J Allergy Clin Immunol* 1992;90:335-339.

9. Jacobs RL, Rake GW Jr, Fournier DC, et al: Potentiated anaphylaxis in patients with drug-induced beta-adrenergic blockade. *J Allergy Clin Immunol* 1981;68:125-127.

10. Chafee FH: The prevalence of bee sting allergy in an allergic population. *Acta Allergol* 1970;25:292-293.

11. van der Linden PW, Struyvenberg A, Kraaijanhagen RJ, et al: Anaphylactic shock after insect-sting challenge in 138 persons with a previous insect-sting reaction. *Ann Intern Med* 1993;118:161-168.

12. Lockey RF, Turkeltaub PC, Baird-Warren IA, et al: The Hymenoptera venom study I, 1979-1982: demographics and history-sting data. *J Allergy Clin Immunol* 1988;82:370-381.

13. Portnoy JM, Moffitt JE, Golden DB, et al: Stinging insect hypersensitivity: a practice parameter. *J Allergy Clin Immunol* 1999;103:963-980.

14. Hunt KJ, Valentine MD, Sobotka AK, et al: Diagnosis of allergy to stinging insects by testing with Hymenoptera venoms. *Ann Intern Med* 1976;85:56-59.

15. Li JT, Yunginger JW: Management of insect sting hypersensitivity. *Mayo Clin Proc* 1992;67:188-194.

16. Hamilton RG, Wisenauer JA, Golden DB, et al: Selection of Hymenoptera venoms for immunotherapy on the basis of patient's IgE antibody cross-reactivity. *J Allergy Clin Immunol* 1993;92:651-659.

17. Sobotka AK, Adkinson NF Jr, Valentine MD, et al: Allergy to insect stings. IV. Diagnosis by radioallergosorbent test (RAST). *J Immunol* 1978;121:2477-2484.

18. Hunt KJ, Valentine MD, Sobotka AK, et al: A controlled trial of immunotherapy in insect hypersensitivity. *N Engl J Med* 1978;299:157-161.

19. Graft DF, Schuberth KC, Kagey-Sobotka A, et al: Assessment of prolonged venom immunotherapy in children. *J Allergy Clin Immunol* 1987;80:162-169.

20. Golden DB, Lawrence ID, Hamilton RH, et al: Clinical correlation of the venom-specific IgG antibody level during maintenance venom immunotherapy. *J Allergy Clin Immunol* 1992;90:386-393.

21. Golden DB, Valentine MD, Kagey-Sobotka A, et al: Regimens of Hymenoptera venom immunotherapy. *Ann Intern Med* 1980;92:620-624.

22. Committee on Insects, American Academy of Allergy, Asthma and Immunology: Position statement: the discontinuation of Hymenoptera venom immunotherapy. *J Allergy Clin Immunol* 1998;101:573-575.

23. Reisman RE: Duration of venom immunotherapy: relationship to the severity of symptoms of initial insect sting anaphylaxis. *J Allergy Clin Immunol* 1993;92:831-836.

14

Anaphylaxis

naphylaxis, which is derived from the Latin words *ana* (against) and *phylaxis* (protection), is a term that was coined by Portier and Richet at the turn of the century to describe an immune reaction that was harmful, rather than protective, to the host. Today, anaphylaxis is used to describe a sudden, immunologically mediated reaction to a foreign substance that produces a severe and potentially life-threatening reaction. Clinical manifestations of anaphylaxis vary widely, but typically involve the cardiovascular system, respiratory tract, gastrointestinal system, skin, and central nervous system (Table 1).[1,2] Cardiovascular manifestations of anaphylaxis include tachycardia, decreased cardiac contractility, capillary leakage, and hypotension. Respiratory signs and symptoms range from mild rhinorrhea or watering of the eyes to laryngospasm, laryngeal edema, or severe bronchospasm. Abdominal pain is also common, especially with ingested allergens, and may be accompanied by either vomiting or diarrhea. Uterine contractions can also be triggered by anaphylaxis, producing severe abdominal pain. Skin manifestations include hives, urticaria, generalized flushing, or pruritus. Disorientation, panic, and loss of consciousness indicate central nervous system involvement. In fatal cases

Table 1: Clinical Manifestations of Anaphylaxis

Organ system	Signs and symptoms
Skin	Flushing Urticaria Angioedema Pruritus
Gastrointestinal	Abdominal pain Vomiting Diarrhea Uterine contractions
Respiratory	Wheezing Hoarseness of the voice Stridor Coughing
Neurologic	Disorientation Seizures
Cardiovascular	Tachycardia Hypotension

of anaphylaxis, petechial hemorrhages and laryngeal edema have been recorded. However, there are no specific findings in up to one half of cases, probably reflecting the role of shock and the rapidity of death.

Although most anaphylactic reactions occur soon after exposure to an inciting agent, there are three patterns of systemic anaphylaxis.[3] Unimodal anaphylaxis usually begins rapidly, and the clinical manifestations are usually short-lived. Bimodal anaphylaxis can also begin within minutes of exposure, but 1 to 8 hours after a transient clinical improvement, the reactions return. Finally, protracted anaphylaxis can begin suddenly or gradually, but the clinical manifestations are prolonged, sometimes requiring hours or even days of intense resuscitation. With these three different clinical presentations in mind, it is important that a patient who has suffered an anaphylactic episode be observed for an adequate length of time.[3,4] For milder reactions, this is typically 3 to 4 hours, but patients who have had severe reactions should be hospitalized overnight for observation.

Several mechanisms may produce general systemic reactions. These can be classified in terms of the underlying pathophysiology (Table 2). Proteins or smaller molecules (haptens) that are bound to native proteins can bind to allergen-specific immunoglobulin E (IgE) present on the surface of mast cells, triggering a type I hypersensitivity reaction.[5] Most authors classify reactions that are mediated by allergen-specific IgE as *anaphylactic*, while clinically indistinguishable reactions that occur via other mechanisms are termed *anaphylactoid* reactions.[6,7] Examples of anaphylactoid reactions include immune complex activation of complement during administration of human serum proteins such as intravenous γ-globulin or direct triggering of mast cell mediator release by substances such as radiocontrast materials, opiates, and dextran.[8] Nonsteroidal anti-inflammatory medications, such as aspirin, may produce anaphylactoid reactions in some patients through a mechanism involving mast cell activation and production of leukotrienes.[9,10]

Diagnosis

Anaphylaxis is a clinical diagnosis. In most cases, there is a clear history of a sudden and sometimes catastrophic reaction after the administration of an inciting agent (Table 1). In some cases, however, the agent is never identified, and a significant number of patients have recurrent anaphylaxis of idiopathic origin.[11,12] Because anaphylaxis can evolve rapidly, patients must be reassessed frequently, especially in terms of the respiratory and cardiovascular systems. Laboratory evaluation is usually neither helpful nor necessary during the acute reaction, but increased blood levels of tryptase, a marker of mast cell activation, are present in 25% to 50% of

Table 2: Classification of Anaphylactic and Anaphylactoid Reactions

IgE mediated (type I hypersensitivity)
- Food—peanuts, tree nuts, seafood, eggs
- Drugs—penicillin, cephalosporins, insulin, serum, allergenic extracts
- Stinging insect (Hymenoptera) venom—bees, yellow jackets, wasps, fire ants
- Other—latex, seminal proteins

Direct stimulation of mast cell degranulation
- Drugs—opiates, vancomycin
- Radiocontrast material
- Physical stimuli—exercise, cold
- Idiopathic

Increased leukotriene synthesis
- Aspirin and other nonsteroidal anti-inflammatory drugs

Complement activation
- Transfusion reaction
- Immunoglobulin

Other
- Sulfite-induced bronchospasm
- Scombroid fish poisoning

cases and may retrospectively confirm the diagnosis of anaphylaxis.[13,14] Because many cases of anaphylaxis are initially unwitnessed, health-care providers should check the patient for a bracelet or necklace bearing information about allergies and carefully review the medical record for any record of allergies or systemic reactions.

Treatment

Treatment of anaphylactic reactions is based on the same principles, regardless of the precipitating cause.[12] Treatment should be tailored to the severity of the reaction and to the organ systems involved (Table 3). Mild anaphylactic reactions with manifestations limited to the skin should be treated with antihistamines such as diphenhydramine (Benadryl®) or hydroxyzine (Atarax®, Vistaril®). These antihistamines have a quick onset of action and provide effective relief of urticaria, pruritus, and flushing. Nevertheless, patients who present with cutaneous reactions should be monitored closely for signs of respiratory or cardiovascular compromise.

The initial treatment of choice for anaphylactic reactions involving organs other than the skin is the rapid intramuscular administration of epinephrine (Ana-Kit®, EpiPen®).[15] This is especially important because surveys of fatal or near-fatal anaphylactic reactions have identified the delayed use of epinephrine as a poor prognostic factor.[16,17] The intramuscular route for administering epinephrine is preferred over subcutaneous injection because of more rapid absorption.[18]

In addition to administration of epinephrine, patients should be placed in Trendelenburg's position, if tolerated, to maximize blood flow to the vital organs, and all patients with respiratory compromise should promptly receive supplemental oxygen. Nebulized albuterol (Proventil®, Ventolin®) should also be administered (in addition to subcutaneous epinephrine) to patients with bronchospasm. Oral or parenteral corticosteroids administered early in therapy may help to prevent prolonged or recurrent symptoms. These measures, plus close observation, adequately treat most cases of anaphylaxis.

Additional measures are required for patients who present with severe anaphylaxis or do not respond to initial treatment. Epinephrine administration should be repeated every 10 to 20 minutes as needed to treat persistent hypo-

Table 3: Treatment of Anaphylaxis

Remove the stimulus for anaphylaxis, if possible

- Stop infusion of offending drug or blood products
- For stings or injections, consider tourniquet proximal to site to retard absorption*

Perform rapid assessment

    Airways

    Breathing

    Circulation

    Vital Signs

Activate emergency medical systems for transfer, if necessary

Treatment of mild cutaneous reactions

- Antihistamine
  - Diphenhydramine 1 mg/kg PO q 4-6 h
- Observation

Treatment of severe cutaneous reactions or reactions with extracutaneous manifestations

Initial treatment:

- Administer O_2
- Epinephrine 1:1,000 0.01 mL/kg (maximum 0.3 mL) intramuscularly
- Trendelenburg positioning (if tolerated)
- Antihistamine
  - Diphenhydramine 1 mg/kg PO, IV, or IM

---

* Tourniquets should be tight enough to impede venous return without obliterating distal pulses.

Initial treatment: *(continued)*
- Nebulized β-adrenergic agonist as needed for bronchospasm
- Corticosteroid
  - Prednisone 1 mg/kg PO q 6 h, or
  - Methylprednisolone 1-2 mg/kg IV q 6 h

For severe symptoms or inadequate response:
- Repeat epinephrine 1:1,000 0.01 mL/kg (maximum 0.3 mL) subcutaneously every 10-20 minutes, *and*

For respiratory symptoms:
- Continue O_2
- Continue nebulized β-agonists for lower airway obstruction
- Intubation for upper airway obstruction or impending respiratory failure

For cardiovascular symptoms:
- Rapid administration of isotonic intravenous fluids
- Sympathomimetic drug via continuous infusion (eg, dopamine)
- Application of medical antishock trousers
- Glucagon 0.03-0.1 mg/kg/dose (max 1 mg/dose) intravenously q 20 min

Reassess condition frequently
- Consider hospitalization

Consider referral to an allergist for prevention of future episodes tension or respiratory compromise. For persistent broncho-spasm, nebulized β-agonists should be continued, and intravenous aminophylline and corticosteroids may be added. Intubation may be required for patients with significant laryngeal edema who do not respond to subcutaneous epinephrine or who have impending respiratory failure.

All patients with significant cardiovascular compromise should have a large-gauge intravenous catheter inserted quickly. Hypotension should be aggressively treated with subcutaneous epinephrine, rapid infusion of intravenous fluid such as normal saline or Ringer's lactate, and Trendelenburg positioning (if tolerated). In patients who are refractory to epinephrine and fluid resuscitation, vasopressors such as dopamine, ephedrine, or norepinephrine given via a constant intravenous drip can be useful in restoring blood pressure.[1,6,7] Medical antishock trousers have also been used successfully to treat refractory hypotension associated with anaphylaxis.[19] Any patient with severe respiratory or cardiovascular compromise should be hospitalized, and monitoring in an intensive care unit should be considered.

Special measures may be needed to treat anaphylaxis in patients taking β-adrenergic blockers such as propranolol (Inderal®) because these patients can develop refractory hypotension and bradycardia.[20] Epinephrine is still first-line therapy in these patients,[20,21] although its use in the presence of β-adrenergic blockade may lead to undesirable effects such as peripheral and coronary vasoconstriction from unopposed α-adrenergic stimulation. Glucagon may be helpful in treating cardiovascular symptoms in patients receiving β-blockers because it exerts inotropic and chronotropic effects via a nonadrenergic mechanism.[20] In addition, atropine (0.3 to 0.5 mg subcutaneous or intramuscular every 10 minutes to a maximum of 2 mg) can be used to treat bradycardia in the presence of β-adrenergic blockade, although atropine does not improve inotropy.[20]

It is important to identify the agent responsible for triggering the anaphylactic episode so that adequate preventive measures can be followed. If the cause of a systemic reaction is unclear, or if preventive therapy is possible, referral to an allergist is strongly recommended.

Prevention

As is the case with most serious medical disorders, the most effective treatment for anaphylaxis is prevention (Table 4). Although most cases of anaphylaxis are unforeseen, a disturbing number of serious allergic reactions are caused by repeated exposure to a known allergen.[4,22,23] While it seems that avoiding a known food or drug allergen would be straightforward, in practice, it may be difficult. For example, in a recent survey of fatal or near-fatal reactions to foods, each of the patients had reacted to the same food previously and was making a conscious effort to avoid the food.[4] Many of the accidental exposures occurred away from home, where there is less control of the ingredients of meals. Patients should be taught to carefully read labels of food ingredients and be especially vigilant when eating away from home.

Multiple safeguards are required to adequately protect drug- or latex-allergic patients from reexposure to allergens. Hospital charts should be flagged, and it is prudent to also notify the hospital and outpatient pharmacy of medication allergies to increase the level of safety. Hospital, outpatient clinic, and ancillary service (phlebotomy, radiology) protocols should be developed ahead of time to ensure the safety of these patients.[24]

Patients who are at risk for repeat anaphylaxis should have an emergency action plan to prepare for the potential of future reactions. This is of primary importance for children with food allergy who are enrolled in school or day care.[25] The plan should include emergency contact telephone numbers, prescriptions with instructions to administer oral antihistamines for cutaneous reactions, and epinephrine to treat systemic reactions involving other organ systems. Unfortunately, surveys have indicated that

Table 4: Preventive Measures

Avoid reexposure to the inciting agent

- Medications
  - Flag the medical record
  - Notify the patient's pharmacy
- Foods
  - Totally exclude the offending food protein from the diet
  - Teach the patient to read product labels
- Stinging insects
  - Avoid eating outdoors during warm-weather months
  - Avoid wearing perfumes outdoors
  - Avoid wearing floral colors during warm-weather months
- Latex
  - Avoid latex exposure in the medical setting
  - Provide lists of home products that contain latex
- Physical stimuli
  - Cold
  - Exercise

epinephrine is often not administered to children who are experiencing anaphylaxis, even when it is available in the home or at school.[26] Moreover, although most paramedics can administer epinephrine, basic-level emergency medical technicians, who are often the first to respond to an emergency, are not permitted to administer epinephrine in many states.[27] Until these regulations are revised, it is critical that high-risk children and adults carry epinephrine autoinjectors and know how and when to use them. Patients should be instructed to seek medical care immediately if

Prepare the patient for accidental exposures to inciting agents

- Oral antihistamine administration for reactions that are limited to the skin
- Epinephrine for self-administration (EpiPen® or Ana-Kit®) for more severe reactions

Preventive therapy

- Immunotherapy for stinging insect hypersensitivity
- Aspirin desensitization
- Oral desensitization for penicillin (or other medication) allergy
- Prophylactic medication regimens

Medical alert bracelets

epinephrine use is necessary, given the short half-life of this medication.

Several modes of therapy have been shown to be effective in preventing anaphylactic reactions. Immunotherapy for stinging insect hypersensitivity is 97% effective at preventing systemic reactions upon re-sting.[28] Effective desensitization regimens have also been established for many medications, including penicillin, sulfonamides, and aspirin.[5] Patients with exercise-induced anaphylaxis should exercise only with a partner and should be aware of early

Table 5: Prophylactic Medications for Patients Allergic to Radiocontrast Material or Latex

The following doses are recommendations and should be adjusted according to a patient's health status, concurrent medications, and disease state. Choose either oral or intravenous regimen (not both):

1. Oral regimen

Medication

Diphenhydramine (Benadryl®)*

Prednisone (Deltasone®) or prednisolone (Pediapred®, Prelone®)

2. Intravenous regimen

Medication

Diphenhydramine*

Methylprednisolone (Medrol®, Solu-Medrol®)

*An H_2-receptor antagonist such as cimetidine (Tagamet®) can also be administered 1 h before the procedure if combined H_1 and H_2 blockade is desired.

warning signs so that severe episodes can be avoided. Prophylactic use of antihistamines may decrease the severity or frequency of idiopathic or exercise-induced anaphylaxis in some patients, but responses vary considerably. While

222

Pediatric dose	Adult dose
1 mg/kg PO 1 h preoperatively (maximum 50 mg/dose)	50 mg PO 1 h preoperatively
1.0 mg/kg PO 13, 7, and 1 h preoperatively (maximum 50 mg/dose)	50 mg PO 13, 7, and 1 h preoperatively

Pediatric dose	Adult dose
1 mg/kg IV 1 h preoperatively (maximum 50 mg/dose)	50 mg IV 1 h preoperatively
1 mg/kg IV 13, 7, and 1 h preoperatively (maximum 50 mg/dose)	50 mg IV 13, 7, and 1 h preoperatively

undergoing radiologic procedures, patients with anaphylactoid reactions to radiocontrast material may be pretreated with an antihistamine along with a corticosteroid (Table 5) to decrease the frequency and severity of reactions.[29] Use of contrast material with low osmolality may be better tolerated by patients with a history of adverse reactions to standard media, although premedication is still advisable.[29] Similar regimens have been recommended for latex-allergic patients undergoing surgical procedures, although the use of prophylactic medications is *not* a substitute for avoiding contact with latex through the use of nonlatex gloves and other medical supplies.[24]

Finally, bracelets or necklaces containing information about allergies may be advisable for patients with a history of systemic reactions. These aids can help health-care providers arrive at a diagnosis quickly so that appropriate treatments can be started without delay.

Summary

Systemic anaphylaxis is relatively rare, but the appropriate initial management of the medical emergency greatly increases the chances for a full recovery. Primary health-care providers and emergency department physicians are most likely to encounter patients with acute anaphylaxis and need to be familiar with its signs and symptoms as well as with resuscitation measures. It is important to identify the precipitating agent for anaphylaxis so that preventive measures can be taken to reduce the risk of future reactions.

References

1. Ritter M, Lemanske RF Jr: Anaphylaxis. In: Zimmerman J, Fuhrman B, eds. *Pediatric Critical Care*. St. Louis, CV Mosby, 1992, pp 1043-1052.

2. Pumphrey RS, Roberts IS: Postmortem findings after fatal anaphylactic reactions. *J Clin Pathol* 2000;53:273-276.

3. Stark BJ, Sullivan TJ: Biphasic and protracted anaphylaxis. *J Allergy Clin Immunol* 1986;78:76-83.

4. Sampson HA, Mendelson L, Rosen JP: Fatal and near-fatal anaphylactic reactions to food in children and adolescents. *N Engl J Med* 1992;327:380-384.

5. Adkinson NF Jr: Drug allergy. In: Middleton E Jr, Reed CE, Ellis EF, et al, eds. *Allergy: Principles and Practice*. St. Louis, Mosby-Year Book, 1998, pp 1212-1224.

6. Winbery SL, Lieberman PL: Anaphylaxis. In: Virant SL, ed. *Systemic Reactions*. Philadelphia, WB Saunders, 1995, pp 447-475.

7. Bochner BS, Lichtenstein LM: Anaphylaxis. *N Engl J Med* 1991;324:1785-1790.

8. VanArsdel PP Jr: Pseudoallergic drug reactions. *Immunol Allergy Clin North Am* 1991;11:635-644.

9. Israel E, Fischer AR, Rosenberg MA, et al: The pivotal role of 5-lipoxygenase products in the reaction of aspirin-sensitive asthmatics to aspirin. *Am Rev Respir Dis* 1993;148:1447-1451.

10. Fischer AR, Rosenberg MA, Lilly CM, et al: Direct evidence for a role of the mast cell in the nasal response to aspirin in aspirin-sensitive asthma. *J Allergy Clin Immunol* 1994;94:1046-1056.

11. Patterson R, Stoloff RS, Greenberger PA, et al: Algorithms for the diagnosis and management of idiopathic anaphylaxis. *Ann Allergy* 1993;71:40-44.

12. Joint Task Force on Practice Parameters, American Academy of Allergy, Asthma and Immunology, American College of Allergy, Asthma and Immunology, and the Joint Council of Allergy, Asthma and Immunology: The diagnosis and management of anaphylaxis. *J Allergy Clin Immunol* 1998;101:S465-S528.

13. Tanus T, Mines D, Atkins PC, et al: Serum tryptase in idiopathic anaphylaxis: a case report and review of the literature. *Ann Emerg Med* 1994;24:104-107.

14. Schwartz LB, Bradford TR, Rouse C, et al: Development of a new, more sensitive immunoassay for human tryptase: use in systemic anaphylaxis. *J Clin Immunol* 1994;14:190-204.

15. AAAI Board of Directors: The use of epinephrine in the treatment of anaphylaxis. *J Allergy Clin Immunol* 1994;94:666-668.

16. Yunginger JW, Sweeney KG, Sturner WQ, et al: Fatal food-induced anaphylaxis. *JAMA* 1988;260:1450-1452.

17. Frazier CA, Wynn SR, Munoz-Furlong A, et al: Anaphylaxis at school: etiologic factors, prevalence, and treatment. *Pediatrics* 1993;91:516.

18. Simons FE, Roberts JR, Gu X, et al: Epinephrine absorption in children with a history of anaphylaxis. *J Allergy Clin Immunol* 1998;101:33-37.

19. Oertel T, Loehr MM: Bee-sting anaphylaxis: the use of medical antishock trousers. *Ann Emerg Med* 1984;13:459-461.

20. Lieberman PL: Anaphylaxis and anaphylactoid reactions. In: Middelton E Jr, Reed CE, Ellis EF, et al, eds. *Allergy: Principles and Practice*. St. Louis, Mosby-Year Book, 1998, pp 1079-1092.

21. Toogood JH: Risk of anaphylaxis in patients receiving beta-blocker drugs. *J Allergy Clin Immunol* 1988;81:1-5.

22. Bock SA, Atkins FM: The natural history of peanut allergy. *J Allergy Clin Immunol* 1989;83:900-904.

23. Gern JE, Yang E, Evrard HM, et al: Allergic reactions to milk-contaminated "nondairy" products. *N Engl J Med* 1991; 324:976-979.

24. Slater JE: Latex allergy. *J Allergy Clin Immunol* 1994; 94:139-149.

25. AAAAI Board of Directors: Anaphylaxis in schools and other child-care settings. *J Allergy Clin Immunol* 1998;102:173-176.

26. Gold MS, Sainsbury R: First aid and anaphylaxis management in children who are prescribed an epinephrine autoinjector device (EpiPen). *J Allergy Clin Immunol* 2000;106:171-176.

27. Goldhaber SZ: Administration of epinephrine by emergency medical technicians. *N Engl J Med* 2000;342:822.

28. Hunt KJ, Valentine MD, Sobotka AK, et al: A controlled trial of immunotherapy in insect hypersensitivity. *N Engl J Med* 1978;299:157-161.

29. Bush WH, Swanson DP: Radiocontrast. In: Virant SL, ed. *Systemic Reactions*. Philadelphia, WB Saunders, 1995, pp 597-612.

15

Complications of Allergic Diseases

C hronic cellular inflammation, mucus hyperse
cretion, and mucosal edema usually accompany
respiratory allergies, and when they do, they can
produce several complications, including sinusitis and otitis media. The infectious complications result from compromised local immunity, which in the upper and lower
respiratory tracts greatly depends on adequate drainage of
respiratory air spaces. Drainage of the respiratory sinuses
and the middle ear occurs through narrow passageways that
are easily occluded by allergen-induced mucosal edema.
Obstruction of the eustachian tube or sinus ostia produces
pooling of secretions that can lead to facial pressure, ear
pain, and, eventually, bacterial upper respiratory infections.

While inflammation clearly exerts mechanical effects on
upper respiratory air spaces, evidence also suggests that preexisting inflammation, such as that which accompanies respiratory allergies, leads to increased adherence of pathogens
to respiratory epithelial cells. For example, treatment of endothelial or epithelial cells with inflammatory cytokines
such as tumor necrosis factor-α (TNF-α) or interleukin-1
(IL-1) promotes binding of *Streptococcus pneumoniae* to the
cell membrane and internalization of bacteria into the cell.[1]
Because these cytokines are increased in allergic airways,

these findings suggest a second mechanism linking allergy with an increased risk for bacterial respiratory infections.

Nasal polyposis, although not strongly associated with respiratory allergy per se, is strongly associated with aspirin hypersensitivity and with chronic sinusitis in allergic and nonallergic individuals. This chapter examines the diagnostic and therapeutic approaches to otitis media, sinusitis, and nasal polyposis.

Otitis Media

Nearly all children develop otitis media in the first 6 years of life, but a subset of these children have recurrent infections that may interfere with hearing, school attendance, and overall health. Several epidemiologic factors have been linked to an increased risk of otitis media, including bottle feeding, low socioeconomic status, cigarette smoke, day-care center attendance, genetic predisposition, and viral infection. The role of allergy in the pathogenesis of otitis media has not been clearly defined. Allergy has been implicated as an epidemiologic risk factor for otitis media in some studies but not others.[2-4] Convincing data, however, indicate that allergen exposure produces eustachian tube dysfunction and that histamine levels are increased in serous middle ear effusions.[5] With this in mind, most investigators have concluded that respiratory allergy is an important risk factor in a subset of children with recurrent otitis media.

Although the microbiology of otitis media (Table 1)[6] has not changed in recent years, therapeutic strategies for it are in a state of flux because of the recent emergence of multiple-drug-resistant bacteria such as *Streptococcus pneumoniae*.[7] In an effort to curtail overuse of antibiotics, which is believed to accelerate the emergence of resistant bacteria, middle ear pathology may be arbitrarily classified as either *acute* or *secretory* otitis media. Acute otitis media is defined as the presence of a middle ear effusion and either concurrent ear pain or evidence of marked in-

Table 1: Microbiology of Acute Otitis Media

- *Streptococcus pneumoniae*
- *Haemophilus influenzae*
- *Moraxella catarrhalis*
- Rhinovirus
- Respiratory syncytial virus

flammation, such as redness or bulging of the tympanic membrane. This process is usually caused by infection with encapsulated bacteria and should be treated with an antibiotic, many of which have proven efficacy for otitis media (Table 2). The choice of antibiotic should be based on several factors, including microbiology, cost, regional patterns of antibiotic susceptibilities, and individual histories of drug allergies or intolerance. Risk factors for antibiotic resistance include attendance at day-care facilities, age less than 2 years, and recent antibiotic treatment.[8] The Centers for Disease Control has formulated recommendations for initial antibiotic therapy of acute otitis media (Table 3). Amoxicillin (Amoxil®, Wymox®) remains an effective and cost-conscious treatment for otitis media in most geographic locations, although a higher dose (80 mg/kg/d) may be required to ensure the eradication of resistant *S pneumoniae*.[8,9] Tympanocentesis and culture of the middle ear fluid can also be used in refractory cases to guide the selection of additional antibiotics.[8,9]

In contrast, secretory otitis media, which may result from eustachian tube dysfunction or may follow treatment of acute otitis media, is defined as middle ear effusion without ear pain or marked local inflammation. In the past, some experts recommended that secretory otitis media be treated aggressively with prolonged courses of antibiotics.

Table 2: Antimicrobial Therapy for Otitis Media and Sinusitis in Children*

Medication	How supplied	Dose
Penicillins		
amoxicillin (Amoxil®, Wymox®)	125 or 250 mg/5 mL 125 or 250 mg chewable tabs	40-80 mg/ kg/day in 3 divided doses
amoxicillin/ clavulanate** (Augmentin®)	125/31, 200/29, 250/62, or 400/58 mg/5 mL 125/31, 200/29, 250/62, or 400/58 mg chewable tabs	40 mg/kg/day in 3 divided doses or 45 mg/kg/day in 2 divided doses (based on amoxicillin component)
Cephalosporins		
loracarbef (Lorabid®)	100 or 200 mg/mL	30 mg/kg/day in 2 divided doses
cefixime (Suprax®)	100 mg/5 mL	9 mg/kg/day in 1 dose

* Duration of therapy: 7-10 days for otitis media, 10-21 days for sinusitis. Children weighing >40 kg should be dosed according to adult guidelines (Table 5).

** Note that Augmentin® chewable tablets contain less clavulanate than Augmentin® tablets, which should only be used by children who weigh >40 kg.

Medication	How supplied	Dose
Cephalosporins *(continued)*		
cefuroxime axetil (Ceftin®)	125 mg/5 mL	30 mg/kg/day in 2 divided doses
cefdinir (Omnicef®)	125 mg/5 mL 300 mg caps	14 mg/kg/day in 1 or 2 divided doses▲
cefpodoxime (Vantin®)	50 and 100 mg/5 mL 100 and 200 mg tabs	10 mg/kg/ in 2 divided doses‡
cefprozil (Cefzil®)	125 and 250 mg/5 mL 250 and 500 mg tabs	15 mg/kg/d in 2 divided doses
ceftibuten (Cedax®)	90 mg/5 mL 400 mg capsules	9 mg/kg/d in single doses
ceftriaxone (Rocephin®)	Vials containing 250 mg, 500 mg, or 1 g	50 mg/kg (not to exceed 1 g) as single IM injection

▲ The recommended duration of treatment for otitis media is 5-10 days for the b.i.d. regimen and 10 days if the medication is administered once daily.

‡ For otitis media, the recommended duration of treatment is 5 days.

(continued on next page)

Table 2: Antimicrobial Therapy for Otitis Media and Sinusitis in Children*
(continued)

Medication	How supplied	Dose
Macrolides		
azithromycin (Zithromax®)	100 or 200 mg/5 mL 250 mg tablets and capsules	100 mg/kg (maximum 500 mg) on day 1, followed by 5 mg/kg (maximum 250 mg) on days 2-5, in single doses
clarithromycin (Biaxin®)	125 or 250 mg/5 mL	15 mg/kg/day in 2 divided doses
Sulfa combinations		
trimethoprim/ sulfamethoxazole (Bactrim®, Septra®)	40 mg TMP + 200 mg SMX per 5 mL	8/40 mg/kg/day in 2 divided doses
erythromycin/ sulfisoxazole (E-Mycin®, ERYC®, Pediazole®)	200 mg erythromycin + 600 mg sulfisoxazole per 5 mL	50/150 mg/kg/day in 4 divided doses

* Duration of therapy: 7-10 days for otitis media, 10-21 days for sinusitis. Children weighing >40 kg should be dosed according to adult guidelines (Table 5).

Because it is now recognized that most cases of secretory otitis media resolve spontaneously, antibiotic therapy is no longer recommended.

For patients with recurrent otitis media, prophylactic antibiotic regimens were used extensively until recently, but these regimens were often only marginally effective and likely contributed to the emergence of drug-resistant organisms. The other treatment option for recurrent otitis media, or for persistent middle ear effusions associated with hearing loss, is the placement of pressure equalization (PE) tubes, which ventilate the middle ear space through the tympanic membrane.[10] PE tubes unquestionably reduce the incidence of otitis media; however, they require a minor surgical procedure and cause local scarring that sometimes leads to complications such as chronic perforation of the tympanic membrane and cholesteatoma. Adenoidectomy also decreases eustachian tube dysfunction in patients with recurrent otitis media and significant adenoid hypertrophy.[11]

Sinusitis

An estimated 25% to 70% of patients with recurrent sinus infections have respiratory allergies, compared with 10% to 20% of the general population.[12-14] In fact, respiratory allergies and viral respiratory infections are the two most important risk factors for the development of acute sinusitis. Mucosal edema and overproduction of respiratory secretions are probably important factors that link respiratory allergy and bacterial sinusitis. Chronic sinusitis can also be caused by fixed obstruction of the sinus drainage tracts, caused by scar tissue, nasal polyps, or anomalies of the nasal bones. The occurrence of both recurrent sinusitis *and* lower respiratory infections strongly suggests the possibility of humoral immune deficiency or cystic fibrosis.[15]

In addition to increasing the risk of bacterial sinusitis, allergy can contribute to local inflammation in patients with fungal sinusitis.[16,17] Patients with allergic fungal sinu-

Table 3: CDC Working Group Treatment Recommendations for Acute Otitis Media*

Antibiotics in prior month	Day 0
No	High-dose amoxicillin;** usual-dose amoxicillin
Yes	High-dose amoxicillin; high-dose amoxicillin/ clavulanate; cefuroxime axetil

CDC = Centers for Disease Control and Prevention

* Recommended drugs are those for which strong evidence for efficacy now exists. Other drugs also may prove efficacious.

** High-dose amoxicillin is 80 to 90 mg per kg per day. High-dose amoxicillin clavulanate is 80 to 90 mg per kg per day of amoxicillin component, with 6.4 mg per kg per day of clavulanate (requires newer formulations or combination with amoxicillin).

sitis do not respond to antibiotic therapy and have positive cultures for fungi from the sinus cavity and evidence of fungus-specific immunoglobulin E (IgE) upon skin testing or radioallergosorbent test.

Symptoms and radiologic changes usually associated with sinusitis can be produced by allergen exposure even without infection. Pelikan conducted a study involving 37 patients with a history of resistant chronic sinusitis in

Clinically defined treatment failure on day 3	Clinically defined treatment failure on days 10-28
High-dose amoxicillin/ clavulanate (Augmentin®);** cefuroxime axetil (Ceftin®); intramuscular ceftriaxone (Rocephin®)[†]	Same as day 3
Intramuscular ceftriaxone;[†] clindamycin;[‡] or tympanocentesis	High-dose amoxicillin/clavulanate; cefuroxime axetil; intramuscular ceftriaxone;[†] or tympanocentesis

[†] Intramuscular ceftriaxone has been documented to be efficacious in acute otitis media treatment failures if 3 daily doses are used.

[‡] Clindamycin is not effective against *Haemophilus influenzae or Moraxella catarrhalis*.

Reprinted from Dowell SF, Butler JC, Giebink GS, et al: Acute otitis media: management and surveillance in an era of pneumococcal resistance—a report from the Drug-Resistant *Streptococcus pneumoniae* Working Group. *Ped Infect Dis J* 1999;18:1-9.

which the patients underwent allergen testing followed by a nasal provocation with allergen.[18] After allergen challenge, 32 patients developed radiologic changes, including increased mucosal edema and opacification of the sinus cavities. These responses were accompanied by symptoms of acute sinusitis, such as increased pressure, headache, and otalgia. These findings demonstrate the contribution of allergen-induced mucosal edema and mucus hypersecretion in the pathogenesis of upper airway symptoms and illustrate the difficulty in evaluating symptoms that suggest infectious sinusitis in allergic patients.

Further evidence of an association between chronic sinusitis and respiratory allergy was provided by a study of 104 patients with chronic sinusitis who were scheduled to undergo endoscopic surgery.[19] Extensive sinus disease, as documented on computed tomography (CT) scan, correlated closely with specific IgE antibodies to inhalant allergens, peripheral eosinophilia, and eosinophilia of nasal mucosal tissue specimens obtained during surgery. These findings provide evidence that unique immunologic mechanisms may be active in the pathogenesis of infectious sinusitis in allergic individuals.

The clinical findings associated with sinusitis differ with age. Typical findings in children include chronic nasal congestion, rhinorrhea, halitosis, fever, and chronic cough.[20,21] Notably absent in most cases of childhood sinusitis are complaints of facial pressure or tenderness to palpation of the sinuses, both of which are relatively common findings in adults. Much of the difficulty in accurately diagnosing sinusitis stems from the fact that pathopneumonic findings of sinusitis, such as a purulent postnasal drip, are found in relatively few patients, and that most of the signs and symptoms of sinusitis are also produced by viral upper respiratory infections or respiratory allergy. The duration and timing of symptoms can be helpful clues: viral upper respiratory infections typically last between 7 to 10 days, while sinus infections are more likely when symptoms endure for longer periods.[20,22] Symptoms that have a seasonal pattern are more likely to be allergic, although secondary sinus infections are common complications of respiratory allergy.

Radiologic evaluation of sinusitis is also imperfect.[23] Sinus radiographs detect only 50% to 70% of bacterial sinus infections that are verified by culture of the maxillary sinuses. CT or magnetic resonance imaging (MRI) scans have a greater sensitivity, but the false-positive rate is also increased, and the cost of CT or MRI scans is difficult to

Table 4: Microbiology of Sinusitis

Organism	Children Acute	Children Chronic	Adults Acute	Adults Chronic
S pneumoniae	+++	+++	+++	+
H influenzae	+++	+++	+++	+
M catarrhalis	+++	+++	++	+
Anaerobes		+	+	+++
S aureus		+	+	++
Fungi		+		+
Viruses	+		+	

+ = reported, ++ = occasional, +++ = common

justify for routine use in primary care medicine. Limited CT scanning of the sinuses, which provides a few key sectional views, is available in some centers and has the advantages of increased sensitivity and relatively low cost. In patients with chronic sinusitis for whom surgery is being considered, CT or MRI scanning is the procedure of choice for defining the anatomy of the ostiomeatal complex.

The microbiology of acute sinusitis is identical to that of acute otitis media (Table 4).[20,21,24,25] *S pneumoniae, Haemophilus influenzae,* and *Moraxella catarrhalis* are the bacteria most frequently recovered from maxillary sinus aspirates from children and adults with acute sinusitis. In contrast, chronic sinusitis in adults is more likely to be caused by anaerobic bacteria, *Staphylococcus aureus,* or fungi.

Treatment of sinusitis should be tailored to the individual, depending on the patient's age, presence of chronic sinus disease, and whether there are predisposing factors such as allergy (Figure 1).[12,20,22,25,26] Suggested antibiotics for sinusitis in children and adults are listed in Tables 2 and 5, respec-

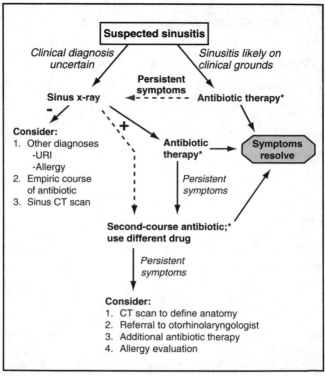

Figure 1: Overview of medical therapy for sinusitis. * See Tables 2 and 4 for suggested antibiotics for use in children and adults with sinusitis. Topical nasal corticosteroid sprays (see Chapter 6, Table 3) may also be beneficial in some patients with sinusitis.

tively. The individual choice depends on the immediate history of antimicrobial therapy, drug allergies, and cost considerations. Although most patients with sinusitis show clinical improvement after 3 or 4 days of therapy with an appropriate antibiotic, we recommend that antibiotic therapy be continued for at least 2 weeks to decrease the chance of relapse. If symptoms are not improved, the diagnosis of sinusitis should be reconsidered, and a sinus radiograph should be ordered if this was not done previously (Figure 1). Because antibiotic-resistant bacteria are becoming increasingly common, a second course of a different antibiotic should be prescribed if sinusitis is confirmed. Further lack of improvement should trigger consultation with an otorhinolaryngologist for consideration of sinus aspiration and culture. A sinus CT scan at this stage is usually advisable to determine whether anatomic abnormalities of the sinus drainage tracts exist.

Several adjuvant therapies, including use of antihistamines, decongestants, topical vasoconstrictors, mucolytic agents, and topical nasal corticosteroids, are widely used for treating sinusitis, despite a paucity of data regarding efficacy.[26] Topical vasoconstrictors cause rebound congestion if used for more than 4 or 5 days, and their chronic use should be avoided. One controlled study examined the effects of a topical nasal corticosteroid (flunisolide [Nasalide®, Nasarel®]) as an adjuvant to antibiotic therapy to treat sinusitis.[27] Nasal mucosal edema was slightly less and patient satisfaction was slightly higher in the flunisolide-treated group, although the relapse rates were similar in both groups (26% vs 35% for placebo-treated subjects). Additional studies are required to establish whether there are subsets of patients with sinusitis that derive greater benefits from adjunctive use of topical corticosteroids.

The epidemiologic association between sinusitis and respiratory allergy suggests that patients with recurrent sinusitis should be evaluated for respiratory allergies. Achieving adequate control of allergen-induced mucosal edema and hypersecretion of mucus by allergen avoidance, medications, and, in selected cases, immunotherapy, helps reduce chronic respiratory symptoms and the frequency of sinusitis.[13,28]

Nasal Polyps

Nasal polyps, which are outgrowths of nasal mucosa, are usually located on the lateral wall of the nose. The characteristic appearance of a nasal polyp is best described as round or

Table 5: Treatment of Sinusitis in Adults*

Medication	How supplied
Acute sinusitis	
amoxicillin (Amoxil®)	250 or 500 mg caps
amoxicillin/clavulanate (Augmentin®)	250-125, 500-125, or 875-125 mg tabs**
azithromycin (Zithromax®)▲	250 mg caps or tabs
cefixime (Suprax®)▲	200 or 400 mg tabs
cefuroxime axetil (Ceftin®)	125, 250, or 500 mg tabs
clarithromycin (Biaxin®)	250 or 500 mg tabs 500 mg extended-release tabs
loracarbef (Lorabid®)	200 or 400 mg caps
trimethoprim/ sulfamethoxazole (Bactrim®)▲	80/400 or 160/800 mg tabs
gatifloxacin (Tequin®)	200 and 400 mg tabs
levofloxacin (Levaquin®)	250 and 500 mg tabs
moxifloxacin (Avelox®)	400 mg tabs
cefdinir (Omnicef®)	300 mg tabs
cefprozil (Cefzil®)	250 and 500 mg tabs

* The duration of therapy should be 2-3 weeks (except 5 days for azithromycin) to decrease the likelihood of relapse; however, if there is no clinical response after 1 week, consider switching medications.

** The clavulanate dose is 125 mg for either the 250- or 500-mg tablets; therefore, the 500-mg dose should *not* be given as two 250-mg tablets.

▲ Medications that are widely used but not approved by the Food and Drug Administration for the treatment of sinusitis.

Dose

500 mg PO q 8 h

250-500 mg PO t.i.d
500-875 mg PO b.i.d.

500 mg PO on day 1, then 250 mg PO on days 2-5

400 mg PO q day

250-500 mg PO b.i.d.

500 mg PO q 12 h, or 1 g extended-release tabs PO q 24 h

400 mg PO q 12 h
160/800 mg PO q 12 h

400 mg q day
500 mg q day
400 mg q day
600 mg/d in 1 or 2 divided doses
250-500 mg q 12 h

(continued on next page)

Table 5: Treatment of Sinusitis in Adults
(continued)

Medication	How supplied
Chronic sinusitis***	
amoxicillin/clavulanate	250-125 or 500-125 mg tabs
ciprofloxacin (Cipro®)	250, 500, or 750 mg tabs
clarithromycin	250 or 500 mg tabs
clindamycin (Cleocin®)	75, 150, or 300 mg caps
doxycycline (Doryx®, Vibramycin®)	50 or 100 mg caps or tabs
metronidazole (Flagyl®, Protostat®)	250, 375, or 500 mg tabs or caps
penicillin V (Pen-Vee® K)	250 or 500 mg tabs

*** Combination therapy to cover aerobes and anaerobes is often used. Treatment failures are common, even if appropriate antibiotics are chosen, when sinus drainage is blocked.

pear-shaped, pale, and gelatinous, and resembling a peeled grape in texture. Most nasal polyps originate in the ethmoid sinus but may occur in other sinuses as well. Nasal polyps are most common among men over the age of 40 and especially in those individuals with aspirin-sensitive asthma.[29] The main morbidity associated with nasal polyps is sinusitis, but it is not clear whether the recurrent sinusitis is the stimulus for polyp growth or vice versa. Polyps are unusual in patients with uncomplicated allergy, except in allergic individuals with recurrent sinusitis. The occurrence of nasal polyps in childhood strongly suggests the diagnosis of cystic fibrosis.

The histology of nasal polyps is remarkable only for normal tissue constituents with chronic cellular inflammation. A polyp consists of an epithelial layer surrounding

Dose

500 mg PO q 8 h (based on amoxicillin component)

500-750 mg PO q 12 h

500 mg PO q 12 h

150-300 mg PO t.i.d. or q.i.d.

100 mg PO q 12 h on day 1, then 50 mg PO q 12 h

375-500 mg PO t.i.d. or q.i.d.

500 mg PO q.i.d.

edematous fibrous tissue infiltrated with eosinophils, mast cells, and lymphocytes.[30,31] Increased levels of immunoglobulin in nasal polyp fluid are further evidence of local activation of the immune system.

Signs and symptoms associated with nasal polyposis include nasal congestion, rhinorrhea, sneezing, postnasal drip, facial pain, and loss of sense of smell (anosmia). The clinical presentation thus resembles that of allergic rhinitis. Despite the lack of association with allergy, patients with nasal polyps have an increased incidence of bronchial hyperresponsiveness and asthma, especially patients with both asthma and aspirin sensitivity.

Treatments for nasal polyps include application of topical corticosteroid sprays or surgical removal.[29,32] Approximately 80% of patients with nasal polyps experience significant improvement after using topical corticosteroid sprays (see Chapter 6, Table 3). Injecting corticosteroid directly into the polyp was a widely used and effective treatment for nasal polyps, but because of several reports of unilateral visual loss following this procedure, this can no longer be recommended.

Patients who have an incomplete response to corticosteroids, indicated by persistent symptoms or recurrent sinus infections, should be referred to an otorhinolaryngologist for polypectomy. Polypectomy usually produces dramatic symptom relief, but the polyps almost invariably return over time. Postoperative use of topical corticosteroid sprays may decrease the regrowth of polypoid tissue.

References

1. Cundell DR, Gerard NP, Gerard C, et al: *Streptococcus pneumoniae* anchor to activated human cells by the receptor for platelet-activating factor. *Nature* 1995;377:435-438.

2. Tainio VM, Savilahti E, Salmenpera L, et al: Risk factors for infantile recurrent otitis media: atopy but not type of feeding. *Pediatr Res* 1988;23:509-512.

3. Fireman P: Eustachian tube obstruction and allergy: a role in otitis media with effusion? *J Allergy Clin Immunol* 1985;76: 137-140.

4. Eiriksson TH, Sigurgeirsson B, Ardal B, et al: Cord blood IgE levels are influenced by gestational age but do not predict allergic manifestations in infants. *Pediatr Allergy Immunol* 1994;5:5-10.

5. Fireman P: The role of antihistamines in otitis. *J Allergy Clin Immunol* 1990;86:638-641.

6. Casselbrant ML, Mandel EM, Kurs-Lasky M, et al: Otitis media in a population of black American and white American infants, 0-2 years of age. *Int J Pediatr Otorhinolaryngol* 1995;33:1-16.

7. Paradise JL: Managing otitis media: a time for change. *Pediatrics* 1995;96:712-715.

8. Pichichero ME: Acute otitis media. Part II. Treatment in an era of increasing antibiotic resistance. *Am Fam Physician* 2000; 61:2410-2416.

9. Dowell SF, Butler JC, Giebink GS, et al: Acute otitis media: management and surveillance in an era of pneumococcal resistance—a report from the Drug-Resistant *Streptococcus pneumoniae* Working Group. *Ped Infect Dis J* 1999;18:1-9.

10. Casselbrant ML, Kaleida PH, Rockette HE, et al: Efficacy of antimicrobial prophylaxis and of tympanostomy tube insertion for prevention of recurrent acute otitis media: results of a randomized clinical trial. *Pediatr Infect Dis J* 1992;11:278-286.

11. Tuohimaa P, Palva T: The effect of tonsillectomy and adenoidectomy on the intra-tympanic pressure. *J Laryngol Otol* 1987;101:892-896.

12. Furukawa CT: The role of allergy in sinusitis in children. *J Allergy Clin Immunol* 1992;90:515-517.

13. Spector SL: The role of allergy in sinusitis in adults. *J Allergy Clin Immunol* 1992;90:518-520.

14. Savolainen S: Allergy in patients with acute maxillary sinusitis. *Allergy* 1989;44:116-122.

15. Gern JE, Lederman HM: Immunodeficiency. In: Noe DA, Rock RC, eds. *Laboratory Medicine: The Selection and Interpretation of Clinical Laboratory Studies.* Baltimore, Williams and Wilkins, 1994, pp 254-275.

16. deShazo RD, Swain RE: Diagnostic criteria for allergic fungal sinusitis. *J Allergy Clin Immunol* 1995;96:24-35.

17. Corey JP, Delsupehe KG, Ferguson BJ: Allergic fungal sinusitis: allergic, infectious, or both? *Otolaryngol Head Neck Surg* 1995;113:110-119.

18. Pelikan Z, Pelikan-Filipek M: Role of nasal allergy in chronic maxillary sinusitis—diagnostic value of nasal challenge with allergen. *J Allergy Clin Immunol* 1990;86:484-491.

19. Newman LJ, Platts-Mills TA, Phillips CD, et al: Chronic sinusitis. Relationship of computed tomographic findings to allergy, asthma, and eosinophilia. *JAMA* 1994;271:363-367.

20. Wald ER: Sinusitis in children. *N Engl J Med* 1992;326:319-323.

21. Wald ER, Milmoe GJ, Bowen A, et al: Acute maxillary sinusitis in children. *N Engl J Med* 1981;304:749-754.

22. Druce HM: Diagnosis of sinusitis in adults: history, physical examination, nasal cytology, echo, and rhinoscope. *J Allergy Clin Immunol* 1992;90:436-441.

23. Diament MJ: The diagnosis of sinusitis in infants and children: x-ray, computed tomography, and magnetic resonance imaging. Diagnostic imaging of pediatric sinusitis. *J Allergy Clin Immunol* 1992;90:442-444.

24. Evans FO Jr, Sydnor JB, Moore WE, et al: Sinusitis of the maxillary antrum. *N Engl J Med* 1975;293:735-739.

25. Gwaltney JM Jr, Scheld WM, Sande MA, et al: The microbial etiology and antimicrobial therapy of adults with acute community-acquired sinusitis: a fifteen-year experience at the University of Virginia and review of other selected studies. *J Allergy Clin Immunol* 1992;90:457-462.

26. Spector SL, et al: Parameters for the diagnosis and management of sinusitis. *J Allergy Clin Immunol* 1998;102:S107-S144.

27. Meltzer EO, Orgel HA, Backhaus JW, et al: Intranasal flunisolide spray as an adjunct to oral antibiotic therapy for sinusitis. *J Allergy Clin Immunol* 1993;92:812-823.

28. Mabry RL: Allergic and infective rhinosinusitis: differential diagnosis and interrelationship. *Otolaryngol Head Neck Surg* 1994;111:335-339.

29. Slavin RG: Nasal polyps and sinusitis. *JAMA* 1997;278:1849-1854.

30. Stoop AE, van der Heijden HA, Biewenga J, et al: Eosinophils in nasal polyps and nasal mucosa: an immunohistochemical study. *J Allergy Clin Immunol* 1993;91:616-622.

31. Stoop AE, van der Heijden HA, Biewenga J, et al: Lymphocytes and nonlymphoid cells in human nasal polyps. *J Allergy Clin Immunol* 1991;87:470-475.

32. Lanza DC, Kennedy DW: Current concepts in the surgical management of nasal polyposis. *J Allergy Clin Immunol* 1992;90:543-546.

16

Treatment Options for Allergy and Asthma

The best way to treat an allergic disease is to identify the offending allergen and remove it from the environment to prevent future reactions from occurring. Sometimes this goal is achieved, but more often, patients continue to be exposed to low levels of allergen or have intermittent and accidental exposures to allergens, such as often happens with food allergy. Consequently, although there is considerable value in identifying specific allergens and in striving to prevent contact with those allergens, other means of therapy are needed to treat acute symptoms, to reduce underlying chronic allergic inflammation, and to reduce the risk of future allergic reactions. This is especially true in treating diseases such as atopic dermatitis and nonallergic asthma, in which the inflammatory mechanisms are similar to allergy but specific allergens are usually not implicated in the disease process. This chapter examines the roles of allergen avoidance, medications, immunotherapy, and other precautionary measures in the treatment of asthma and atopic disorders (Table 1).

Allergen Avoidance

In addition to causing seasonal and perennial rhinoconjunctivitis, overwhelming evidence indicates that respirato-

Table 1: Overview of Therapy for Allergic Diseases

Allergen avoidance

Symptomatic medications

- Antihistamines
- Decongestants
- β-adrenergic agonists
- Anticholinergics

Preventive medications

- Mast cell stabilizing agents
- Corticosteroids
- Leukotriene modifiers

Allergen desensitization

Precautionary measures

- Epinephrine for self-administration
- Indicate allergies on hospital and pharmacy records
- Medical alert bracelets

ry allergies are a significant factor in the pathogenesis of asthma, especially in children. Limiting exposure to relevant indoor allergens can lead to reductions in asthma symptoms, bronchial hyperresponsiveness, and use of asthma medications.[1] Therefore, patients with significant asthma should be evaluated for respiratory allergies, and the asthma treatment plan should always include detailed instructions to the patient, child, and family to help minimize exposure to relevant allergens (Table 2). Avoidance measures are especially effective in decreasing exposure to indoor allergens such as pet dander, house dust mite, and mold. Avoiding contact with cat or dog allergens is straightforward in principle: find another home for the pet.

Table 2: Control of Indoor Allergens

House dust mite
- Encase mattress in an airtight cover
- Encase pillows, or wash weekly in hot water
- Wash blankets and bed linens in hot (>130°F) water every 10-14 days
- Avoid upholstered furniture
- If feasible, remove carpets in the bedroom
- If possible, keep humidity <50%

Pets
- Remove from the house (especially if contributing to asthma)

Mold
- Use a dehumidifier in the basement
- Remove carpets laid over concrete
- If possible, keep humidity <50%
- Fix leaks in roof, bathrooms, etc.

Some patients with allergic rhinitis may be willing to tolerate significant upper airway symptoms to keep a beloved pet, but when the animal contributes to asthma, removing the pet from the home is clearly the best choice in light of the morbidity and even mortality associated with asthma. Unfortunately, reports that washing pets or treating them with acepromazine can reduce their allergen shedding and thus limit allergy symptoms have not been substantiated.[2]

House dust mites are arachnids that are too small to be seen with the naked eye. These highly allergenic creatures cohabitate with humans, with little regard for whether a home is clean or dirty. They eat skin scales and are thus found in high concentrations in bedding, upholstered furniture, and carpets. Successful methods of controlling dust mite allergen concentrations include encasing mattresses and pillows in plastic, washing bed covers and linens in hot (>130°F) water, and removing carpets and upholstered furniture.[3] Acaricides such as malathion also reduce mite numbers, but few people are willing to use insecticides indoors. Tannic acid solutions denature mite proteins and render them less allergenic; however, tannic acid can stain furniture and carpets, and clinical benefits after treatments with it have not been demonstrated.[4] Maintaining indoor humidity at less than 50% is an effective way to control dust mites and molds.[3] Important sources of indoor mold include damp carpets, especially carpet laid on concrete slab, and construction materials that are water damaged from leaks or flooding. Faulty ventilation systems can also increase exposure to allergenic molds.

Controlling exposure to outdoor allergens such as pollens and molds is difficult, but a few measures can be helpful. Closing the windows and using either air conditioning or a high-efficiency air filter help limit indoor mold spore and pollen counts. Limiting outdoor exercise during peak allergen seasons, especially in the morning hours, can also be beneficial.

Allergen avoidance is the only effective treatment for food allergy.[5] Patients or parents must be taught to carefully read the labels of prepared foods, and they must be able to recognize all forms of the allergenic protein. Although avoidance is simple in principle, accidental ingestion of foods identified as allergenic is common, especially when eating away from home.[6,7] Parents sending children with food allergy to school or day care for the first time should explain to teachers the dietary restrictions and contingency plans for the treatment of accidental ingestion of an allergen.[8] The Food Allergy & Anaphylaxis Network (10400 Eaton Place, Suite 107, Fairfax, VA 22030, 703-691-3179, http://www.foodallergy.org) is a parent-run organization that is a valuable source of information about living with food allergy.

Antihistamines

Antihistamines block the interaction between histamine and histamine-specific receptors. H_1-receptor antagonists are the most useful drugs for treating allergic symptoms, although the addition of H_2-antihistamines may provide some additional relief for patients with chronic urticaria. Because histamine is one of many mediators involved in allergic inflammation, antihistamines usually provide only partial relief from allergic symptoms. In general, antihistamines are fairly effective for treatment of urticaria, sneezing, itching, and rhinorrhea, but they have relatively little effect on congestion,[9] which is one of the most troublesome symptoms of allergic rhinitis. Some antihistamines produce bronchodilation, but its effect is too small to be clinically significant in patients with asthma. Antihistamines do not cause mucus plugging in the lower airway and can be used safely in patients with asthma.

First-generation antihistamines are effective histamine-receptor blockers, but produce clinically apparent sedation in about one third of users. Studies using neural psychological testing or monitoring of brain waves have demonstrated that subtle central nervous system effects can be demonstrated in a much greater fraction of subjects taking standard antihistamines.[10,11] Furthermore, tests in a sophisticated driving simulator suggest that effects of standard doses of diphenhydramine (Benadryl®) on driving performance are similar to those caused by a blood alcohol level of 0.1 mg/mL.[12] Second-generation antihistamines, which are lipophobic and do not cross the blood-brain barrier (with the exception of cetirizine [Zyrtec®]), retain potent antihistaminic effects, have relatively long half-lives, and produce sedation in very few individuals (Chapter 6, Table 3).[9] Although antihistamines are generally safe, cardiac arrhythmias can occur with overdoses of certain antihistamines or with standard doses if administered to patients with liver disease, to patients taking medications such as erythromycin and ketoconazole (Nizoral®) that slow hepatic clearance, or to patients with prolonged QTc interval.[9] Fexofenadine (Allegra®), loratadine (Claritin®), cetirizine, and acrivastine (Semprex-D®) do not produce cardiac side effects because they do not prolong the QTc interval.[9]

Topical antihistamines, such as levocabastine (Livostin®), can be used on an as-needed basis for the symptomatic relief of allergic rhinitis and conjunctivitis. In addition to blocking the H_2-receptor, some of the topical H_1 blockers (eg, azelastine [Astelin®], ketotifen [Zaditor®]) may have anti-inflammatory effects to relieve allergic symptoms, including inhibition of eosinophil recruitment and mast cell and eosinophil activation.[13,14]

Decongestants and Vasoconstrictors

α-Adrenergic agonists have potent vasoconstrictive effects when administered either orally or topically and are widely used as adjunctive medications for allergic rhinoconjunctivitis. Antihistamines are often combined in drug mixtures with decongestants, which may counteract the sedative effect of antihistamines to some degree and potentiate the decongestive effects of the antihistamine. Unfortunately, oral decongestants sometimes produce side effects that limit their clinical utility, including tremor, insomnia, nervousness, and restriction of urinary flow in males.[15] Topical α-adrenergic agonists such as oxymetazoline (Afrin®) or phenylephrine (Neo-Synephrine®) are potent vasoconstrictors, but these medications produce rebound congestion if used for more than a few days and so are unsuitable for treating patients with chronic allergic rhinitis. Most nonprescription cold and allergy preparations containing phenylpropanolamine (PPA) were recently withdrawn from the market in response to a public health warning by the US Food and Drug Administration (FDA). Preliminary analysis of a clinical research study revealed that use of PPA was associated with a small but significant increase in the incidence of stroke.

Bronchodilators
Drug delivery systems

Aerosol delivery of medications would seem to be ideally suited for asthma therapy because it maximizes drug delivery to the small airway while minimizing the systemic effects of medications. Although there are definite theoretic advantages to drug delivery via inhalation, clinical responses to aerosolized medications vary widely. The principal reason for these inconsistent responses is that the mechanics of breathing (eg, inspiratory flow, duration of breath-holding) greatly affect the amount of medicine that reaches the lungs.

Inhaled medications are usually administered either by nebulizer or pressurized metered-dose inhaler (MDI), although some medications are also available in dry powder inhalers. The optimum particle size for lower airway deposition is 1 mm to 5 mm. Larger droplets are likely to stay in the upper airway.[16] MDIs generate relatively smaller 'respirable' particles compared to nebulizers, which may explain why nebulizer doses of β-agonists must be 3 to 10 times larger to achieve the same degree of bronchodilation. MDIs have the additional advantages of being more portable and quicker to use, and they cost 50% to 75% less per treatment than nebulizers. Although nebulizers have traditionally been used in medical facilities for treating acute asthma, MDIs provide bronchodilation that is faster and of equal or greater magnitude, although larger than standard doses may be required.[17]

MDIs that contain chlorofluorocarbons (CFCs) contribute to the depletion of stratospheric ozone. As a result of the consequent health hazards, CFCs have been internationally banned. Although a temporary medical exemption has been granted, MDIs with CFC propellants will eventually have to be replaced with alternative aerosol products. The first non-CFC albuterol MDI was recently approved. This MDI is driven by an alternate propellant using hydrofluoroalkane (HFA-134a), which does not deplete ozone.

Patients should be counseled that the new HFA MDI may feel different because it generates a less forceful aerosol plume, but it actually does a better job of delivering asthma medications to the lung.[18]

Unfortunately, many patients do not use MDIs correctly (Chapter 7, Table 5) and thus do not derive full benefit from the medications contained within them. Spacer devices can improve the efficacy of inhaled medications in patients who are unable to master correct inhaler technique.[19] These devices work by trapping most of the large aerosol droplets while holding the smaller particles in a reservoir until they are inhaled. Some brands of spacers, such as the Aerochamber®, can be equipped with variable-size masks suitable for use by young children. For older children, spacers equipped with mouthpieces are preferred because the nose may filter out particles that would otherwise be deposited in the lung. In addition to improving drug delivery to the lower airways, the use of a spacer with inhaled corticosteroids (ICS) also reduces the incidence of side effects such as oral candidiasis and hoarseness.

Epinephrine and β-adrenergic agonists

Epinephrine is a catecholamine that has long been used to relieve acute symptoms of allergy. Because epinephrine is inactivated in the gastrointestinal tract, it must be either inhaled or injected. The potent α-adrenergic (increased heart rate, stroke volume, and vascular tone) and β-adrenergic (bronchodilator) effects of epinephrine make it the drug of choice for treating anaphylactic reactions. Delayed use of epinephrine in anaphylactic reactions has been associated with a poorer outcome.[6,7] Epinephrine for self-administration should be prescribed for patients at risk for repeated anaphylaxis (eg, food allergy, idiopathic anaphylaxis) and may also be useful for patients with a history of severe paroxysmal asthma. Injectable epinephrine is available in several forms; however, the EpiPen® (0.3 mg) and EpiPen® Jr. (0.15 mg) are especially easy to use, which is a distinct advantage in an emergency. Medical alert bracelets are also advisable for patients who have experienced anaphylactic reactions in the past.

Inhaled selective β_2-agonists, which produce longer-lasting bronchodilation with less discomfort, have largely replaced injected epinephrine in the management of acute asthma (see Chapter 8). The availability of β_2-agonists in multiple forms (short-, intermediate-, and long-acting) and delivery systems (MDIs, nebulizer solutions, oral liquids and tablets, respirable powders) gives them wide clinical versatility. Short-acting β_2-agonists are the most effective medications for relieving bronchospasm and are the drugs of choice for treating acute asthma symptoms and exacerbations and for preventing exercise-induced bronchospasm. All patients with asthma, regardless of severity, should have access to a short-acting β_2-agonist at all times.[20] Paradoxically, the rapid onset of action and potent bronchodilator activity may lead to deterioration of asthma disease control if the patient uses β-agonists to the exclusion of anti-inflammatory medications, which do not produce any immediate positive feedback. Therefore, the increasing frequency of β_2-agonist use should be considered an indicator of inadequate disease control and a signal for the need for a medical evaluation. Side effects of selective β_2-agonists include tremor, tachycardia, and increased anxiety, but these occur infrequently when β_2-agonists are administered via inhalation.

Levalbuterol (Xopenex®), which is the R-isomer of albuterol, has recently been approved for the treatment of asthma in adults, and safety and efficacy have recently been demonstrated in children.[21] The S-isomer of albuterol, which is not present in levalbuterol, does not bind to β_2-adrenergic receptors but may contribute to some of the side effects of albuterol (Proventil®, Volmax®). Because the R-isomer is the active component of albuterol, levalbuterol is effective at a lower dose than racemic albuterol. For example, 0.63 mg levalbuterol causes bronchodilation that is similar to 2.5 mg albuterol but with fewer side effects.[22] Therefore, levalbuterol would seem to be a reasonable alternative in patients in whom albuterol (or other short-acting β-agonists) is effective but causes significant side effects (eg, tremor). The reduced side effect profile of levalbuterol may be especially apparent during treatment of status asthmaticus, which may require high-dose and/or continuous β_2-agonist therapy.

Long-acting β_2-agonists such as salmeterol (Serevent®) and formoterol (Foradil®) are best used as adjuncts to anti-inflammatory medications to control persistent asthma.[20,23] For example, in patients who continue to have chronic asthma symptoms despite the use of low-dose ICS, adding salmeterol to the regimen can produce better control of symptoms than is achieved by increasing the dose of ICS.[20] Neither medication, however, should be used to treat persistent asthma without concurrent anti-inflammatory therapy such as ICS. In addition, salmeterol should not be used for the relief of acute asthma symptoms because of the relatively slow onset of action compared to short-acting β_2-agonists such as albuterol.

Theophylline

Theophylline is a methylxanthine drug that produces bronchodilation by inhibiting phosphodiesterase (PDE), causing increases in smooth-muscle cyclic adenosine monophosphate (AMP). Several studies suggest that theophylline has anti-inflammatory effects, including inhibition of inflammatory-cell mediator release. Theophylline is available in liquid, beaded capsule, and tablet forms, including several sustained-release formulations that may be given at 8-hour to 24-hour intervals. Aminophylline, the amino-salt of theophylline, is administered intravenously.

Theophylline is a safe and effective bronchodilator at serum concentrations of 5 µg/mL to 15 mg/mL. Other beneficial effects of theophylline include attenuation of the early- and late-phase response to allergen, corticosteroid sparing, and improved exercise tolerance.[24] When compared to β_2-agonists, theophylline has a slower onset of action and a lower peak effect, making it less suitable for acute therapy.

Serum levels of theophylline are influenced by a number of variables, including age, diet, disease states, drug inter-

Table 3: Theophylline: Common Drug Interactions*

Medications that decrease serum theophylline levels

- Carbamazepine
- Phenytoin
- Phenobarbital
- Rifampin

Medications that increase serum theophylline levels

- Macrolide antibiotics
- Cimetidine
- Ciprofloxacin
- Oral contraceptives
- Zileuton
- Disulfiram
- Propranolol
- Mexiletine
- Allopurinol
- Verapamil

Medications with accentuated side effects when administered with theophylline

- Cetirizine
- Ephedrine
- Tetracycline

---

* This list is not all inclusive; consult the medical literature before prescribing other medications along with theophylline.

actions, and hepatic clearance, all of which contribute to the complexity of using this medication.[24] For example, tobacco and marijuana smoking increase theophylline metabolism, while febrile illnesses and high carbohydrate diets significantly decrease theophylline metabolism. Potential drug interactions require that the dose of theophylline be adjusted accordingly (Table 3). Because of the variability of theophylline metabolism, as well as its narrow therapeutic index, serum concentrations of theophylline should be monitored periodically.

Unfortunately, theophylline may produce a number of dose-related side effects, such as nausea, irritability, and insomnia. The frequency and severity of these side effects can be minimized by initiating therapy with a low dose of theophylline and gradually increasing the dose to achieve therapeutic serum concentrations.[24] Of concern to parents and teachers is the suggestion that chronic use of theophylline might adversely affect school performance, although recent studies have not substantiated this association. For example, controlled studies of children taking theophylline for long-term asthma management have found no effects on either behavior or performance on standardized achievement tests.[25]

Anticholinergics

Anticholinergic medications such as atropine inhibit the muscarinic effects of acetylcholine, producing bronchodilation. Ipratropium bromide (Atrovent®) is a closely related quaternary ammonium compound that also causes bronchodilation, but because it is poorly absorbed into the systemic circulation, it has fewer side effects than atropine. Because the bronchodilation produced by anticholinergic medications has a slower onset of action and a smaller peak effect compared to β-adrenergic agonists, their use in asthma is limited. Their role is best defined for use in chronic obstructive pulmonary disease. Ipratropium is available as an MDI, solution for nebulization, and a nasal spray. Ipratropium nasal spray acts directly on secretory glands to decrease the production of nasal secretions and has a mild decongestant effect. Ipratropium effectively inhibits rhinorrhea caused by vasomotor rhinitis or the common cold,[26] but its role in the management of allergic rhinitis remains to be determined.

Anti-Inflammatory Medications
Antiallergic medications

Cromolyn sodium and nedocromil sodium (Tilade®) are two structurally distinct asthma medications that have very similar properties. Both medications inhibit inflammatory cell activation, mediator release, early and late allergen-induced bronchoconstriction, and airway hyperresponsiveness. Although cromolyn and nedocromil attenuate exercise- and allergen-induced bronchospasm, they do not have direct bronchodilating effects. Their mechanisms of action are not well understood but probably involve inhibition of chloride channels or neurokinins. Cromolyn is available in several forms: MDI (Intal®), solution for nebulization, nasal spray (Nasalcrom®), and ophthalmic solution (Crolom®). Nedocromil is only available as an MDI, but other forms are forthcoming. A third mast cell stabilizing agent, lodoxamide (Alomide®), has been released as an ophthalmic solution for the treatment of allergic conjunctivitis.

Clinical studies have confirmed that regular use of cromolyn or nedocromil for asthma improves pulmonary function and reduces respiratory symptoms and the use of rescue medications.[27,28] The use of these drugs may be limited because they must be dosed 4 times daily, although the dosing frequency can usually be reduced to t.i.d. or b.i.d. in patients with a good initial response. In children, cromolyn sodium and nedocromil have excellent safety records and can be used to control asthma. Cromolyn nasal spray, which is available over the counter, is somewhat less effective for allergic rhinitis. Cromolyn and lodoxamide eyedrops are effective prophylactic treatments for ocular allergies when used regularly.[29,30]

Corticosteroids

Glucocorticosteroids are the most potent anti-inflammatory agents available for the treatment of allergic inflammation and asthma.[31] Their efficacy is related to many factors, including a diminution in inflammatory cell function and activation, stabilization of vascular leakage, a decrease in mucus production, and an increase in β-adrenergic response.

Unfortunately, chronic administration of oral glucocorticosteroids may result in multiple dose-dependent adverse effects, including hypothalamic pituitary adrenal axis suppression, osteoporosis, posterior subcapsular cataracts, hyperglycemia, hypertension, dermal thinning and striae, and the potential for growth retardation.[31] In addition, although short courses of oral corticosteroids rarely cause serious side effects, corticosteroid therapy may exacerbate preexisting health problems such as hypertension or diabetes. Finally, case reports of fatal varicella infection associated with systemic corticosteroid use in children with asthma suggest a potential danger.[32] As a result, patients who contract varicella during or within 30 days of a course of oral corticosteroid may require additional treatments such as a course of oral acyclovir (Zovirax®). It is also prudent to administer varicella vaccine to children or adults without a history of chickenpox who are likely to require oral corticosteroids for asthma.

Fortunately, because ICS are effective in children and adults, the need for oral corticosteroid regimens has diminished substantially. ICS are the most potent and effective anti-inflammatory therapy available for asthma and have few side effects when used at standard doses. The two most common side effects are hoarseness and oral candidiasis, occurring in less than 10% of patients. The incidence of these side effects is further reduced by using spacer devices and instructing patients to rinse their mouth and gargle after using ICS. It is clear, however, that high-dose ICS (see Chapter 7, Table 6) can cause systemic side effects, especially when high-potency corticosteroids are used.

The potential effects of ICS on growth are of interest to health-care providers caring for children with asthma. Some data suggest that even standard doses of ICS can adversely affect short-term growth in some children,[33] suggesting that individual tolerances to ICS vary considerably. Notably, studies of long-term (>12 months) ICS therapy have generally not found adverse effects on growth.[33-35] These data suggest that ICS can be used safely in children with the following precautions. First, all children requiring prolonged oral or inhaled corticosteroid at any dose should be measured carefully at routine intervals to monitor effects on stature. In addition, once respiratory symptoms are controlled, the dose of corticosteroid should be tapered to the lowest effective dose.

Topical corticosteroid preparations are also the treatment of choice for moderate to severe allergic rhinitis. They relieve a broad range of symptoms, including congestion, which is generally not affected by antihistamine therapy. Prolonged use of topical corticosteroids in the nose or lower airways is safe, as verified by biopsy studies after prolonged (up to 10 years) daily administration of beclomethasone dipropionate (Beconase®, Vancenase®). Side effects associated with topical nasal corticosteroids are uncommon but include nosebleeds and local nasal inflammation. Septal perforations have been reported rarely and are caused by overdosing or improper inhaler technique (see Chapter 6). However, topical corticosteroids in the eye should be used with extreme caution because of the effects on intraocular pressure, the risk of cataracts, and potentiation of ocular infections such as herpes keratitis. Patients who suffer severe rhinoconjunctivitis during the pollen allergy season may benefit significantly by taking a short course of an oral corticosteroid (eg, prednisone 20 mg PO b.i.d. x 5 days in adolescents or adults). This approach provides prompt and dramatic clinical relief and opens the airway so that topical nasal sprays can reach the target tissues.

Leukotriene Modifiers

The leukotrienes are potent inflammatory mediators that contribute to the pathogenesis of asthma and, to a lesser extent, allergic rhinitis. These compounds are synthesized from arachidonic acid in cell membranes through a series of enzymatically-controlled reactions (Figure 1). Leukotriene synthesis and effects of these mediators can therefore be regulated at several points in this process. Compounds (eg, zileuton [Zyflo®]) that inhibit either 5-lipoxygenase or 5-lipoxygenase activating protein (FLAP) prevent synthesis of leukotrienes, while receptor antagonists (zafirlukast

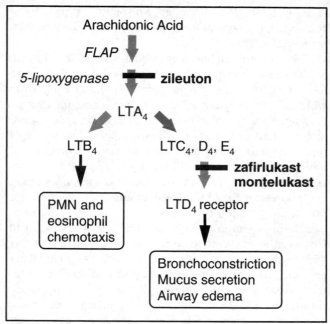

Figure 1: Leukotriene synthesis pathways and activities of leukotriene modifiers.

[Accolate®], montelukast [Singulair®]) block binding of LTC_4, LTD_4, and LTE_4 to their common receptor.

Several observations indicate that leukotrienes are important mediators of inflammation in asthma.[36,37] First, leukotriene synthesis, as measured by urinary LTE_4 excretion, is increased in asthma. Second, inhaled leukotrienes induce a profound and prolonged bronchoconstriction, with LTD_4 exerting greater effects than either LTC_4 of LTE_4. Finally, leukotriene modifiers are effective treatments for asthma.

Although leukotriene synthesis inhibitors and receptor blockers exert their effects through distinct mechanisms, their clinical effects are similar. Both types of leukotriene modifiers produce bronchodilation beginning with the first dose, and chronic use can reduce daytime and nighttime symptoms, produce modest improvements in pulmonary function, and inhibit acute asthma symptoms triggered by exercise, allergen inhalation, and aspirin. In addition, leukotriene modifiers may have anti-inflammatory properties because they reduce circulating eosinophil counts and inhibit allergen-induced eosinophil recruitment to the airway.

Despite their similar effects, a few differences among these leukotriene modifiers can affect their clinical utility. Although these medications share the ease of oral administration and have few side effects, zileuton occasionally produces liver toxicity,[38] and hepatic enzymes (ALT) should be monitored.[19] Zafirlukast and montelukast are less likely to cause hepatic inflammation and do not require monitoring of liver enzymes. Zafirlukast and zileuton are metabolized in the liver: zafirlukast can interfere with warfarin metabolism, and zileuton interferes with warfarin, theophylline, and terfenadine metabolism. In addition, zileuton must be given q.i.d., although patients who have a good initial response may do well on a t.i.d. schedule. Montelukast (once daily) and zafirlukast (b.i.d.) are easier to use because of less frequent dosing, although zafirlukast should be taken on an empty stomach because food interferes with its bioavailability.

As a cautionary note, cases of Churg-Strauss syndrome (pulmonary eosinophilic vasculitis) have been reported in patients with severe asthma soon after starting therapy with zafirlukast or zileuton. It appears, however, that this might not be related to the leukotriene modifier, but rather to the reduction in systemic corticosteroids in a patient with Churg-Strauss syndrome that was previously unrecognized.

Because clinical experience with this new class of medications is limited, their role in controlling asthma symptoms has not been clearly defined. The updated National Heart, Lung, and Blood Institute *Guidelines for the Diagnosis and Management of Asthma*[19] classify these compounds as an alternative *controller* for the treatment of mild persistent asthma. This seems especially appropriate in patients who are unwilling to use ICS. In addition, it is reasonable to consider leukotriene modifiers as a supplement to other asthma controllers to reduce the need for high-dose ICS therapy or in the management of asthma patients with aspirin sensitivity.[36,37]

Clarification of the role of leukotriene modifiers in the treatment of asthma awaits studies that compare these medications head-to-head with conventional asthma controllers, and additional information gathered during real-life use in patients with asthma.

Immunotherapy

Immunotherapy involves injecting gradually increasing amounts of an allergen into a sensitized patient in an effort to induce a state of tolerance to that allergen. Although the precise mechanism underlying the induction of tolerance is unknown, several hypotheses have been advanced. Clinical changes such as reduction in immediate and late-phase reactivity to allergens correspond with a number of immunologic alterations, including a rise in allergen-specific IgG_4 antibodies, decreased allergen-specific IgE, and a shift in T-cell responses away from TH2 and towards a TH1-like cytokine response pattern.[39] Which one of these immunologic changes causes the clinical improvement is uncertain. Regardless of the mechanism, immunotherapy has proven efficacy for the treatment of several allergic disorders, including stinging insect hypersensitivity, allergic rhinoconjunctivitis, and, in some instances, asthma.[40,41]

Immunotherapy for stinging insect hypersensitivity is curative and reduces the incidence of subsequent systemic allergic reactions after a re-sting to that of the general population. Patients receiving immunotherapy for rhinoconjunctivitis usually experience partial relief of symptoms, enabling better symptom control with less medication. Because the combination of allergen avoidance and medications effectively controls allergy symptoms in most patients, most allergists reserve immunotherapy for patients who do not respond favorably to this combination. Whether asthma can be treated with immunotherapy is controversial,[42,43] but most of the evidence indicates that some subgroups of patients are likely to respond. These subgroups include patients with seasonal asthma from pollen allergy and those with mild or moderate asthma and one or two well-defined allergies. Unstable asthma is a contraindication to immunotherapy because of increased risk of anaphylaxis and fatal reactions.

Immunotherapy for food allergy has been carefully evaluated in a large clinical trial.[44] Unfortunately, because of concerns about safety and efficacy, immunotherapy for food allergy cannot be recommended at this time.

New Directions in Medical Therapy

Several innovative treatments for allergic diseases are under investigation. First, the benefits and side effects of corticosteroids are mediated by at least two distinct intracellular mechanisms (transrepression and transactivation). Recognition of these two pathways has raised hopes for the development of *dissociated steroids*, which would cause only transrepression and thus retain efficacy while causing fewer steroid side effects.[45]

Novel approaches to immunotherapy are also being tested. One approach to provide effective immunotherapy with less risk to the patient has been to inject increasing doses of immunogenic peptides, or protein fragments, engineered from major allergens such as *Fel d* 1 (cat) or *Amb a* 1 (ragweed).[46] Theoretically, much larger doses of the allergen can be given because the peptides are too small to cross-link IgE molecules and trigger mast cell mediator release. Finally, injections of a genetically engineered antibody specific for human IgE have been shown to reduce allergen-induced inflammatory responses in animal models and in patients with mild asthma.[47, 48] Time and clinical research will tell whether these approaches will eventually be useful in clinical practice.

References

1. Duff AL, Platts-Mills TA: Allergens and asthma. *Pediatr Clin North Am* 1992;39:1277-1291.

2. Klucka CV, Ownby DR, Green J, et al: Cat shedding of *Fel d* I is not reduced by washings, Allerpet-C spray, or acepromazine. *J Allergy Clin Immunol* 1995;95:1164-1171.

3. Platts-Mills TA, Vaughan JW, Carter MC, et al: The role of intervention in established allergy: Avoidance of indoor allergens in the treatment of chronic allergic disease. *J Allergy Clin Immunol* 2000;106:787-804.

4. Woodfolk JA, Hayden ML, Couture N, et al: Chemical treatment of carpets to reduce allergen: comparison of the effects of tannic acid and other treatments on proteins derived from dust mites and cats. *J Allergy Clin Immunol* 1995;96:325-333.

5. Sampson HA: Food allergy. *JAMA* 1997;278:1888-1894.

6. Sampson HA, Mendelson L, Rosen JP: Fatal and near-fatal anaphylactic reactions to food in children and adolescents. *N Engl J Med* 1992;327:380-384.

6. Yunginger JW, Sweeney KG, Sturner WQ, et al: Fatal food-induced anaphylaxis. *JAMA* 1988;260:1450-1452.

8. Frazier CA, Wynn SR, Munoz-Furlong A, et al: Anaphylaxis at school: etiologic factors, prevalence, and treatment. *Pediatrics* 1993;91:516.

9. Simons FE, Simons KJ: The pharmacology and use of H_1-receptor-antagonist drugs. *N Engl J Med* 1994;330:1663-1670.

10. Bender B, Milgrom H: Neuropsychiatric effects of medications for allergic diseases. *J Allergy Clin Immunol* 1995;95:523-528.

11. Simons FE, Reggin JD, Roberts JR, et al: Benefit/risk ratio of the antihistamines (H_1-receptor antagonists) terfenadine and chlorpheniramine in children. *J Pediatr* 1994;124:979-983.

12. Weiler JM, Bloomfield JR, Woodworth GG, et al: Effects of fexofenadine diphenhydramine and alcohol on driving performance. A randomized, placebo-controlled trial in the Iowa driving simulator. *Ann Intern Med* 2000;132:354-363.

13. Azelastine nasal spray for allergic rhinitis. *Med Lett Drugs Ther* 1997;39:45-47.

14. Kato M, Hattori T, Takahashi M, et al: Eosinophil cationic protein and prophylactic treatment in pollinosis in natural allergen provocation. Br J Clin Pract 1994;48:299-301.

15. Druce HM: Allergic and nonallergic rhinitis. In: Middleton E Jr, Reed CE, Ellis EF, et al, eds. *Allergy: Principles and Practice*. St. Louis, Mosby-Year Book, 1998, pp 1005-1016.

16. Morrow PE: Conference on the scientific basis of respiratory therapy. Aerosol therapy. Aerosol characterization and deposition. *Am Rev Respir Dis* 1974;110:88-99.

17. Kerem E, Levison H, Schuh S, et al: Efficacy of albuterol administered by nebulizer versus spacer device in children with acute asthma. *J Pediatr* 1993;123:313-317.

18. Vanden Burgt JA, Busse WW, Martin RJ, et al: Efficacy and safety overview of a new inhaled corticosteroid, QVAR (hydrofluoroalkane-beclomethasone extrafine inhalation aerosol) in asthma. *J Allergy Clin Immunol* 2000;106:1209-1226.

19. Toogood JH: Helping your patients make better use of MDIs and spacers. *J Respir Dis* 1994;15:151-165.

20. National Asthma Education and Prevention Program, National Heart Lung, and Blood Institute, National Institutes of Health: *Expert Panel Report II: Guidelines for the Diagnosis and Management of Asthma*. Bethesda, U.S. Department of Health and Human Services, 1997.

21. Gawchik SM, Saccar CL, Noonan M, et al: The safety and efficacy of nebulized levalbuterol compared with racemic albuterol and placebo in the treatment of asthma in pediatric patients. *J Allergy Clin Immunol* 1999;103(4):615-621.

22. Nelson HS, Bensch G, Pleskow WW, et al: Improved bronchodilation with levalbuterol compared with racemic albuterol in patients with asthma. *J Allergy Clin Immunol* 1998;102(6 pt 1):943-952.

23. AAAAI Committee on Drugs, American Academy of Allergy, Asthma, and Immunology: Safety and appropriate use of salmeterol in the treatment of asthma. *J Allergy Clin Immunol* 1996;98:475-480.

24. Weinberger M, Hendeles L: Theophylline in asthma. *N Engl J Med* 1996;334:1380-1388.

25. Bender B, Milgrom H: Theophylline-induced behavior change in children. An objective measure of parents' perceptions. *JAMA* 1992;267:2621-2624.

26. Grossman J, Banov C, Boggs P, et al: Use of ipratropium bromide nasal spray in chronic treatment of nonallergic perennial rhinitis, alone and in combination with other perennial rhinitis medications. *J Allergy Clin Immunol* 1995;95:1123-1127.

27. Shapiro GG, Sharpe M, DeRouen TA, et al: Cromolyn versus triamcinalone acetonide for youngsters with moderate asthma. *J Allergy Clin Immunol* 1991;88:742-748.

28. Armenio L, Baldini G, Bardare M, et al: Double-blind, placebo-controlled study of nedocromil sodium in asthma. *Arch Dis Child* 1993;68:193-197.

29. Blumenthal M, Casale T, Dockhorn R, et al: Efficacy and safety of nedocromil sodium ophthalmic solution in the treatment of seasonal allergic conjunctivitis. *Am J Ophthalmol* 1992;113: 56-63.

30. Juniper EF, Guyatt GH, Ferrie PJ, et al: Sodium cromoglycate eye drops: regular versus "as needed" use in the treatment of seasonal allergic conjunctivitis. *J Allergy Clin Immunol* 1994;94:36-43.

31. Schleimer RP: Glucocorticosteroids. Their mechanisms of action and use in allergic diseases. In: Middleton E Jr, Reed CE, Ellis EF, et al, eds. *Allergy: Principles and Practice*. St. Louis, Mosby-Year Book, 1993, pp 893-925.

32. Silk HJ, Guay-Woodford L, Perez-Atayde AR, et al: Fatal varicella in steroid-dependent asthma. *J Allergy Clin Immunol* 1988;81:47-51.

33. Long-term effects of budesonide or nedocromil in children with asthma. The Childhood Asthma Management Program Research Group. *N Engl J Med* 2000;343:1054-1063.

34. Agertoft L, Pedersen S: Effect of a long-term treatment with inhaled budesonide on adult height in children with asthma. *N Engl J Med* 2000;343:1064-1069.

35. Silverstein MD, Yunginger JW, Reed CE, et al: Attained adult height after childhood asthma: effect of glucocorticoid therapy. *J Allergy Clin Immunol* 1997;99:466-474.

36. Horwitz RJ, McGill KA, Busse WW: The role of leukotriene modifiers in the treatment of asthma. *Am J Respir Crit Care Med* 1998;157:1363-1371.

37. Szefler SJ: Leukotriene modifiers: what is their position in asthma therapy? *J Allergy Clin Immunol* 1998;102:170-172.

38. Israel E, Cohn J, Dube L, et al: Effect of treatment with zileuton, a 5-lipoxygenase inhibitor, in patients with asthma. A randomized controlled trial. Zileuton Clinical Trial Group. *JAMA* 1996;275:931-936.

39. Durham SR, Till SJ: Immunologic changes associated with allergen immunotherapy. *J Allergy Clin Immunol* 1998;102:157-164.

40. Weber RW: Immunotherapy with allergens. *JAMA* 1997; 278:1881-1887.

41. Durham SR, et al: Long-term clinical efficacy of grass pollen immunotherapy. *N Engl J Med* 1999;341:468-475.

42. Adkinson NF Jr, Eggleston PA, Eney D, et al: A controlled trial of immunotherapy for asthma in allergic children. *N Engl J Med* 1997;336:324-331.

43. Creticos PS, Reed CE, Norman PS, et al: Ragweed immunotherapy in adult asthma. *N Engl J Med* 1996;334:501-506.

44. Oppenheimer JJ, Nelson HS, Bock SA, et al: Treatment of peanut allergy with rush immunotherapy. *J Allergy Clin Immunol* 1992;90:256-262.

45. Barnes PJ: Anti-inflammatory actions of glucocorticoids: molecular mechanisms. *Clin Sci* 1998;94:557-572.

46. Norman PS: Therapeutic potential of peptides in allergic disease. *Ann Allergy* 1993;71:330-333.

47. Boulet LP, Chapman KR, Côté J, et al: Inhibitory effects of an anti-IgE antibody E25 on allergen-induced early asthmatic response. *Am J Respir Crit Care Med* 1997;155:1835-1840.

48. Fahy JV, Fleming HE, Wong HH, et al: The effect of an anti-IgE monoclonal antibody on the early- and late-phase responses to allergen inhalation in asthmatic subjects. *Am J Respir Crit Care Med* 1997;155:1828-1834.

Index

A

285

theophylline 107, 109, 114, 116, 118, 256-258, 263
thimerosal 74, 163
thiuram 163
thrombocytopenia 31, 188
thrombosis 151
thyroiditis 139, 141
tidal breathing 21
Tilade® 105, 258
tobacco smoke 8, 40, 44, 57, 98, 99, 101, 105
tobacco smoking 27, 257
tolerance 256
Topicort® 158
total serum IgE 51
tourniquets 196, 216
tracheal stenosis 28
tranexamic acid (Cyklokapron®) 150
Trantas' dots 67, 75
trauma 139, 144, 149
treatment failure 235
tree nuts 176, 181, 214
trees 41, 57, 58
tremor 87, 129, 185, 252, 255
Trendelenburg's position 215, 216
trial elimination diet 175
triamcinolone (Aristocort®, Azmacort®, Kenalog®, Nasacort®) 90, 116, 157, 158, 161
Tridesilon® 158
trimethoprim/sulfamethoxazole (Bactrim®, Septra®) 232, 240
tryptase 35, 213
tumor 34

tumor necrosis factor-α (TNF-α) 46, 47, 227
tympanocentesis 229, 235
tyramine 32

U

Ultravate® 158
upper respiratory infection (URI) 22, 85, 101, 227
urinalysis 145
urologic abnormalities 194
urticaria 34-36, 40, 51, 138-140, 142-150, 156, 169, 172, 188, 190, 191, 194, 202-204, 211, 212, 215, 251
US Food and Drug Administration (FDA) 252
uterine contractions 212

V

Vancenase AQ® 90
Vancenase Pockethaler® 90
Vancenase® 261
vancomycin 214
Vantin® 231
varicella 260
vasculitis 144, 148
vasoconstrictors 70, 93, 239, 252
vasomotor rhinitis 85, 93
vasovagal reactions 34
venom 205, 214
venom immunotherapy 202, 208
venom skin tests 208
Ventolin® 105, 129, 130, 215
verapamil 257

NOTES